QUICK GUIDE TO PERIPHERAL VASCULAR STENTING

CHRISTOPHER J. WHITE, MD
CHAIRMAN, DEPARTMENT OF CARDIOLOGY
OCHSNER CLINIC, NEW ORLEANS, LA

STEPHEN R. RAMEE, MD
SECTION HEAD, INVASIVE CARDIOLOGY AND
DIRECTOR CARDIAC CATHETERIZATION LABORATORY
OCHSNER CLINIC, NEW ORLEANS, LA

J. STEPHEN JENKINS, MD
DIRECTOR, DIAGNOSTIC CATHETERIZATION AND
DIRECTOR, EXPERIMENTAL ANGIOPLASTY LABORATORY
OCHSNER CLINIC, NEW ORLEANS, LA

TYRONE J. COLLINS, MD
DIRECTOR, INTERNATIONAL CARDIOLOGY AND
PROGRAM DIRECTOR CARDIOLOGY FELLOWSHIP
OCHSNER CLINIC, NEW ORLEANS, LA

Notice

Treatment recommendations in *Quick Guide to Peripheral Vascular Stenting* are based on practice guidelines, medical literature, and the authors' clinical experience. They are designed as a guide for the management of uncomplicated patients and are not meant as a substitute for sound clinical judgment or individualization of therapy. Though extensive efforts have been made to assure accuracy and completeness, unerring treatment recommendations cannot be guaranteed.

In general, drug indications and dosages listed in this Guide have been recommended in the medical literature and conform to the practices of the general medical community. However, this does not imply approval by the United States Food and Drug Administration (FDA) for their use in the conditions and dosages listed. The use of any drug should be preceded by a careful review of the package insert, which provides indications and dosages as approved by the FDA. As always, it is the obligation of the healthcare professional to keep abreast of the latest developments in the field, including new drug indications and dosages.

Comments and suggestions should be referred to:

Physicians' Press
620 Cherry Street
Royal Oak, Michigan 48073
Tel: (248) 616-3023
Fax: (248) 616-3003

www.physicianspress.com

Printed in the United States of America

ISBN 1-890114-32-4

To my children, Jordan, Jimmy and Casey and my wonderful wife Janet, whose support allows me to do what I do.

Christopher J. White, MD

CONTENTS

Chapter One

INTRODUCTION

INTRODUCTION

Many cardiologists are expanding their practices to include peripheral vascular interventions. This trend will result in improved overall patient care because atherosclerosis is a systemic disease, and patients with coronary disease are at increased risk for other manifestations of occlusive vascular disease. The ability to treat selected patients with percutaneous techniques is cost effective and associated with lower morbidity and mortality than for conventional surgical procedures.

It has been our experience that the technical skills necessary to perform coronary angioplasty are easily transferable to the peripheral procedures. However, an understanding of the natural history of peripheral disease, patient and lesion selection criteria, and the knowledge of other treatment alternatives are essential elements required to perform these procedures safely and effectively. For interventional cardiologists who are inexperienced in the treatment of peripheral vascular disease, appropriate preparation and training and a team approach including involvement of an experienced vascular surgeon are both desirable and necessary before attempting percutaneous peripheral angioplasty.

New stents are appearing at a rapid pace, both balloon expandable and self-expanding. Throughout this book, the Palmaz stent (Cordis/JJIS) has been selected to represent and illustrate the deployment technique for *balloon expandable* stents and the Wallstent (Boston Scientific/Scimed) has been used to illustrate *self-expanding* stent techniques and strategies.

There are inherent advantages for patients when the interventionalist performing the procedure is also the clinician responsible for the pre- and post-procedure care, analogous to the vascular surgeon who cares for patients before and after surgical procedures. Judgments regarding the indications, timing, and risk-to-benefit ratio of procedures are enhanced by a long-term relationship between physician and patient. Finally, in view of the increased incidence of coronary artery disease in patients with atherosclerotic peripheral vascular disease, the participation of a cardiologist in their care seems appropriate.

This text will focus on the three areas of most interest to the cardiologist with an interest in peripheral vascular stent placement, ie. iliac, renal, and carotid artery occlusive disease. The ability of interventional cardiologists to perform peripheral vascular procedures safely and effectively will vary with their individual training and experience. There is no current consensus on the most appropriate credentialing criteria, although several organizations have proposed guidelines.

Another area of confusion and difficulty is that many of the devices necessary for the optimal treatment of peripheral vascular disease have been adapted from other applications and have not yet been approved by the Food and Drug Administration for these specific applications. Nothing in this text should be construed as promotion of unapproved devices for clinical use.

The purpose of this text is to provide interventionalists insight and perspective into what we feel is our current "best" medical practice in a rapidly evolving field of medicine. It is important that each patient's needs be evaluated individually, and that in this rapidly changing field no generalizable treatment recommendations can be made. New stents are appearing at a rapid pace, both balloon expandable and self-expanding. Throughout this book, the Palmaz stent (Cordis/JJIS) has been selected to represent and illustrate the deployment technique for *balloon expandable* stents and the Wallstent (Boston Scientific/Scimed) has been used to illustrate *self-expanding* stent techniques and strategies.

STENTS VERSUS OTHER PERCUTANEOUS MODALITIES

Since the initial work by Dotter in the 1960s and the development of balloon angioplasty by Gruentzig in the 1970s it has become clear that percutaneous intervention is an effective treatment for selected patients with atherosclerotic occlusive peripheral vascular disease. Balloon angioplasty continues to be an effective and valuable tool for many of these patients. However, the limitation of balloon angioplasty includes both acute complications such as dissections which can cause immediate failure of the procedure, and restenosis, the late failure of the procedure. Several classes of devices have been developed to attempt to improve the results of conventional balloon angioplasty. Debulking or tissue removal with lasers and atherectomy devices have been used to improve the ability of the balloon to create a larger neolumen.

While some of these devices continue to be valuable for specific lesion categories, their general application has not been accepted nor justified by clinical data. Stents, on the other hand, have been effective in a variety of clinical situations and vascular beds by: 1) salvaging failed or suboptimal angioplasty results, or 2) by improving the acute gain in luminal diameter following balloon dilation, which results in improved long-term patency of the treated vessel.

There are potential disadvantages associated with stent placement. The additional cost of placing one or more stents can be significant. Whether this cost is justifiable based upon fewer complications and a reduced need for repeat procedures compared to balloon angioplasty remains to be proven. There are complications that are specific to stent placement such as stent embolization and subacute thrombosis that must be considered. Finally, the stent is a foreign body, and as with any implanted foreign body the implanted stent can rarely become the focus of an infection with disastrous clinical consequences.

Peripheral vascular stents have been in clinical use for more than a decade. At this point several issues have become clinically established. In suitable candidates, stents are the most reliable, and safest way to percutaneously open and maintain patency in a stenotic or occluded artery. The technique for optimal stent placement is continuing to evolve with the development of new designs and new strategies for deployment. At present, each patient and each lesion should be evaluated individually for the most appropriate treatment.

Chapter Two

ILIAC ARTERY STENT PLACEMENT

ILIAC ARTERY STENT PLACEMENT

I. Indications for percutaneous therapy of iliac artery obstructive disease

1. To obtain retrograde femoral vascular access in occlusive or stenotic iliac lesions for cardiac diagnostic or therapeutic procedures.
2. To treat iliac artery lesions causing lower extremity and pelvic ischemic symptoms. (**Tables 1 - 3**).
   a. Lifestyle limiting claudication.
   b. Limb-threatening ischemia.
   c. Non-healing ulcers.
   d. Rest pain.
   e. Vascular impotence.

Table 1. Acute limb ischemia assessment (SVS/ISCVS Standards J. Vasc Surg 1986;4:80-94)

Category	Description	Capillary Fill	Muscle Weakness	Sensory Loss	Doppler Signals	
					Arterial	Venous
Viable	No immed risk	Intact	None	None	Audible	Audible
Threatened	Salvageable	Intact Slow	Mild Partial	Sensory Incomplete	Inaudible	Audible
Irreversible	Amputation	Absent Marbling	Profound	Profound	Inaudible	Inaudible

Table 2. Chronic limb ischemia assessment (SVS/ISCVS Standards J. Vasc Surg 1986;4:80-94)

Grade	Category	Clincal Description	Objective Criteria
0	0	Asymptomatic	Normal GXT*
I	1	Mild claudication	Completes GXT, AP 25 to 50 mmHg < BP
I	2	Moderate claudication	Between categories 1 & 3
I	3	Severe claudication	Cannot complete GXT, AP < 50 mm Hg
II	4	Ischemic rest pain	Resting AP < 40 mmHg
III	5	Minor tissue loss	TP < 40 mmHg
III	6	Major tissue loss	Same as category 5

AP = ankle pressure, BP = brachial pressure, TP = toe pressure.

* = five minutes on a treadmill at 2 mph with a 12% incline.

Table 3. Follow-up limb status assessment (SVS/ISCVS Standards J. Vasc Surg 1986;4:80-94)

Changes in limb status graded +3 to -3

+3 = markedly improved, normalized, no symptoms, ABI ≥ 0.9

+2 = moderately improved, one category improved, symptomatic, ABI improved by > 0.10, but not normalized

+1 = minimally improved, no category shift, symptomatic, but ABI < 0.10 improved

0 = no change

-1 = minimally worse, no category shift, ABI > 0.1 decreased

-2 = moderately worse, one category worse, or unexpected minor amputation

-3 = markedly worse, more than one category worse, or unexpected major amputation

ABI = ankle brachial index

II. Indications for iliac artery stent placement

1. Improved acute and long-term patency over balloons. (**Figure 1**)
2. Occlusions.
3. Restenosis lesions.
4. Long lesions.
5. Poor results following balloon angioplasty (PTA).

III. Performing diagnostic aorto-iliac angiography

1. Choosing a vascular access site. (**Figure 2**)

   a. **Brachial artery access:** This is an attractive access site in patients with absent femoral pulses, or in patients with known bilateral iliac artery disease.

Figure 1. Randomized trial of stenting versus angioplasty for iliac arteries.

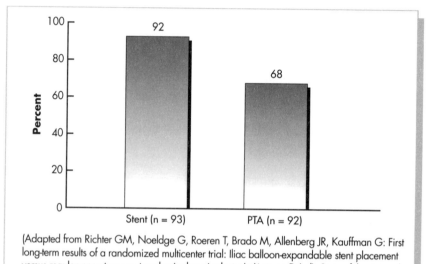

(Adapted from Richter GM, Noeldge G, Roeren T, Brado M, Allenberg JR, Kauffman G: First long-term results of a randomized multicenter trial: Iliac balloon-expandable stent placement versus regular percutaneous transluminal angioplasty. In Lierman D (ed): State of the Art and Future Developments, pp 30-35, Morin Heights, Canada, Polyscience, 1995.)

1) Insert a 6 Fr sheath either percutaneously or by cutdown into the brachial artery.

2) Administer 5,000 IU of heparin.

3) Advance an 0.035-in J-guidewire to the aortic arch.

4) Insert a catheter (pigtail or Judkins-R4) to direct the guidewire over the aortic arch to the descending aorta and place a pigtail catheter at the level of the renal arteries (L1 - L2) in preparation for angiography. Occasionally, a steerable 0.035-in guidewire (Glidewire or Wholey wire) to select the descending aorta.

b. **Contralateral femoral artery access:** This access site is useful when the known or suspected iliac artery lesion is unilateral and located in the distal portion of the external iliac artery.

1) Place a 6 Fr sheath retrogradely into the common femoral artery and give 3,000 IU of heparin.

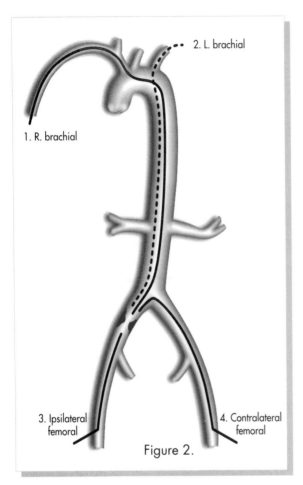

2. L. brachial

1. R. brachial

3. Ipsilateral femoral

4. Contralateral femoral

Figure 2.

Figure 2. Vascular access options. 1. Right brachial access. 2. Left brachial access. 3. Ipsilateral (retrograde) femoral access. 4. Contralateral femoral access.

2) Advance an 0.035-in J-guidewire to the abdominal aorta, and advance a 6 Fr pigtail catheter to the level of the renal arteries (L1 - L2) to perform aorto-iliac angiography.

3) Exchange a 6 Fr internal mammary catheter for the pigtail catheter and select the ostium of the contralateral iliac artery.

c. **Ipsilateral (retrograde) femoral artery access:** This is the most common access site for iliac artery angiography and possible stent placement.

1) Place a 6 Fr sheath into the common femoral artery and administer 3,000 IU of heparin.

2) Cross the lesion with a 0.035-in Wholey wire. *(NB: If the Wholey wire will not cross the lesion, an alternative choice is*

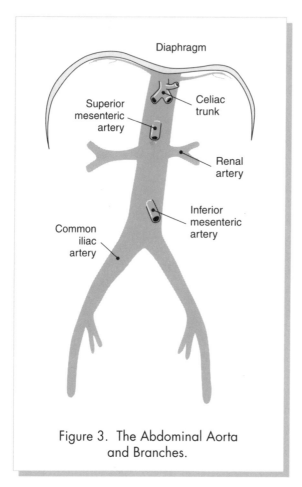

Diaphragm

Superior
mesenteric
artery

Celiac
trunk

Renal
artery

Inferior
mesenteric
artery

Common
iliac
artery

Figure 3. The Abdominal Aorta
and Branches.

an 0.035-in angled Glidewire or a straight extra-stiff Amplatz wire guided by Judkins right coronary catheter.)

3) Once the lesion has been crossed, advance a 6 Fr pigtail catheter to the level of the renal arteries (L1 - L2) in preparation for aorto-iliac angiography.

2. Perform a diagnostic infrarenal aortogram.

a. Position the 6 Fr pigtail catheter so that the sideholes of the catheter are at the level of renal arteries, confirmed with test injections of contrast. *(NB: Placement of the catheter at too high a level will fill the superior mesenteric artery (SMA) which may obscure the ostium of the right renal artery.)* We prefer to use a low osmolar, low viscosity, ionic contrast (Hexabrix-320) or non-ionic contrast for patient comfort. The injection rate using a power injector is 15 cc to 20 cc per second for 2 or 3 seconds.

b. Perform cineangiography with a 9-inch to 16-inch image intensifier at 12.5 frames/sec to 15 frames/sec in the anterior-posterior projection. The table is panned during the injection to visualize the vascular system from the level of the renal arteries to the common femoral arteries. This is an overview angiogram for diagnostic purposes to identify the iliac artery lesion(s) as well as to image the inflow and outflow vessels. *(NB: It is important to visualize the run-off vessels from the target lesion as this will impact on long-term patency of the stent).*

3. Perform selective iliac angiography to better define the lesion.

   a. Selective iliac angiography may be performed from the brachial, contralateral femoral or ipsilateral femoral access site as described above.

      1) Imaging of iliac arteries can be achieved by positioning a 6 Fr pigtail catheter in the terminal aorta, just above the common iliac bifurcation.

      2) From the brachial approach use a long multipurpose A2 catheter which can be directed into the ostium of either iliac artery for selective angiography.

      3) From the contralateral femoral approach, a 6 Fr internal mammary, Simmons, or Cobra catheter may be used to selectively engage the contralateral common iliac artery.

      4) From the ipsilateral femoral approach, a retograde angiogram may be performed through the arterial sheath, or a 6 Fr pigtail catheter may be advanced over a wire across the lesion to obtain a selective antegrade angiographic image of the lesion.

   b. Low osmolar, low visosity, ionic contrast (Hexabrix-320) or non-ionic contrast should be used when performing peripheral angiography.

      1) For terminal aorta injections through the pigtail or multi-

purpose catheter a power injector is used at a rate of 10 cc per second over 2 or 3 seconds. If digital subtraction angiography is the used the contrast injection can be decreased to 10 to 15 cc per second for 1 second. *(NB: For selective angiographic images with end-hole catheters it is necessary to first perform a test injection to make sure the tip of the catheter is free in the lumen of the vessel.)*

2) For selective iliac angiography a power injection of 5 cc per second for 2 or 3 seconds or 10 cc hand injections of contrast are sufficient to opacify the artery.

c. The conventional angiographic view of the iliac artery is in the AP projection. However, given the tortuous course of the vessel over the pelvic brim, an excellent view may be obtained by tilting the image intensifier 20° caudally and 20° medially from the target lesion.

IV. Preparation for iliac artery stent placement

1. Premedicate the patient with 325 mg of aspirin daily.
2. Anticoagulate the patient with 2,500 IU to 5,000 IU of heparin.
3. Vasodilator medications may be helpful in determining the hemodynamic severity of borderline angiographic lesions, or in relieving vessel spasm. Intra-arterial administration of nitroglycerine (0.2 mg) or papaverine (10 mg to 40 mg) may be administered. *(NB: care needs to be taken when administering papaverine that no contrast comes into contact with the drug or a white precipitate will occur.)*
4. Stent delivery catheters/sheaths will vary depending on the choice of vascular access.

    a. From the brachial approach, for delivery of a medium-sized Palmaz stent (expanded diameter 4 mm to 9 mm), an 8 Fr coronary

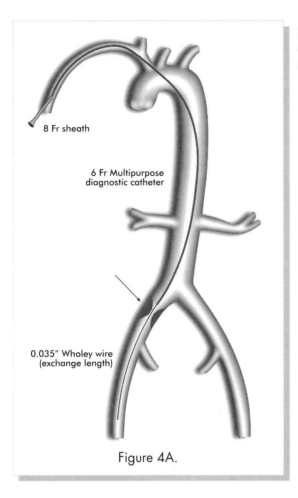

8 Fr sheath

6 Fr Multipurpose
diagnostic catheter

0.035" Wholey wire
(exchange length)

Figure 4A.

Figure 4A. Brachial access: Palmaz iliac artery stent deployment.
  8 Fr sheath in brachial artery, Wholey wire across lesion.

guiding catheter or 6 Fr sheath is required. To deliver a self-expanding Wallstent, a 9 Fr coronary guiding catheter or 7 Fr sheath is required. b. From the contralateral femoral artery approach an 8 Fr "Crossover" guiding catheter or 6 Fr sheath will deliver a deliver a medium sized (expanded diameter 4 mm to 9 mm) Palmaz stent (P104, P154, or P204). A self-expanding Wallstent can be delivered by using a 9 Fr "Crossover" guiding catheter or 7 Fr sheath or a Wallstent may be delivered without a guiding catheter using a short 7 Fr sheath. *(NB: The guiding catheter/sheath allows contrast imaging of the target lesion during stent positioning. If the operator chooses not to use a guiding catheter or sheath, then stent placement must be guided by bony or external landmarks.)*

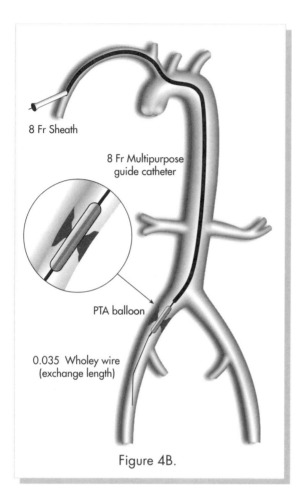

8 Fr Sheath

8 Fr Multipurpose
guide catheter

PTA balloon

0.035 Wholey wire
(exchange length)

Figure 4B.

Figure 4B. Brachial access: Palmaz iliac artery stent deployment. 8 Fr multipurpose guide catheter and predilation balloon.

c. From the ipsilateral (retrograde) femoral artery approach an 8 Fr to 10 Fr long (20 cm to 30 cm) sheath is necessary to deliver a large (8 mm to 12 mm diameter) Palmaz stent (P128, P188 or P308). A long 6 Fr sheath will deliver a medium (4 mm to 9 mm) Palmaz stent (P104, P154, or P204). A conventional 7 Fr sheath is sufficient to deliver a self-expanding Wallstent.

V. Palmaz iliac stent placement from brachial artery access (Figure 4 A - F)

1. Insert an 8 Fr sheath either percutaneously or via cutdown into the brachial artery.
2. Administer 5,000 IU of heparin.

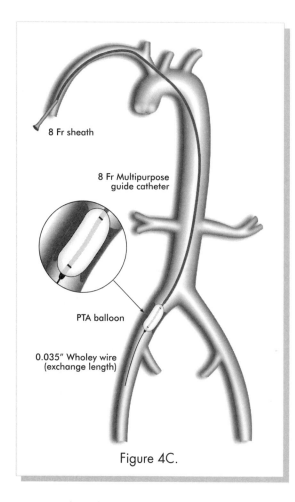

8 Fr sheath

8 Fr Multipurpose
guide catheter

PTA balloon

0.035" Wholey wire
(exchange length)

Figure 4C.

Figure 4C. Brachial access: Palmaz iliac artery stent deployment.

Inflate predilation balloon, exchange for Amplatz extra-stiff wire.

3. Direct a 0.035-in Wholey guidewire (exchange length) over the aortic arch to the descending aorta using either a 6 Fr pigtail or multipurpose catheter to steer the wire to the descending aorta.

4. Exchange the diagnostic 6 Fr catheter for an 8 Fr multipurpose guiding catheter or long 6 Fr sheath and place the wire and guiding catheter into the ostium of the iliac artery.

5. Cross the iliac artery lesion with the steerable, atraumatic 0.035-in Wholey wire. *(NB: If the Wholey wire will not cross the lesion, a 0.035-in angled or straight Glidewire, or an 0.035-in straight extra-stiff Amplatz wire may be used.)*

6. Using test injections of contrast, select the best view, either AP or an angled view (20° caudal and 20° medial), to demonstrate the lesion.

7. Perform a base-line angiogram with the wire across the lesion.

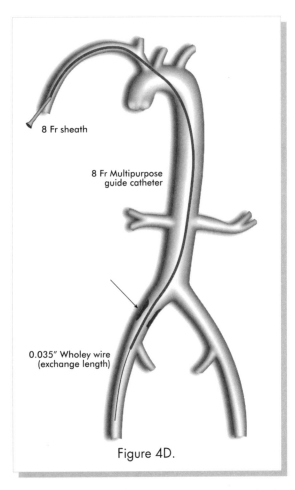

8 Fr sheath

8 Fr Multipurpose
guide catheter

0.035" Wholey wire
(exchange length)

Figure 4D.

Figure 4D. Brachial access: Palmaz iliac artery stent deployment.

Advance guiding catheter across lesion.

8. Measure the reference diameter of the vessel and the lesion length. *(NB: Visual estimation of vessels larger than 4.0 mm is quite variable and overdilation of an artery may lead to rupture or extensive dissection.)*

9. Mark the location of the target lesion with bony landmarks, or with an external radiopaque ruler.

10. Advance a balloon catheter across the lesion, chosen to match the reference artery diameter (1:1), and long enough to cover the lesion.

    a. Remove the Wholey wire from the balloon and measure a hemodynamic gradient across the lesion, using the wire lumen of the balloon catheter and the guiding catheter/sheath.

    b. Advance an exchange length Amplatz extra-stiff wire through the balloon wire lumen to the distal vessels to give added support for stent placement.

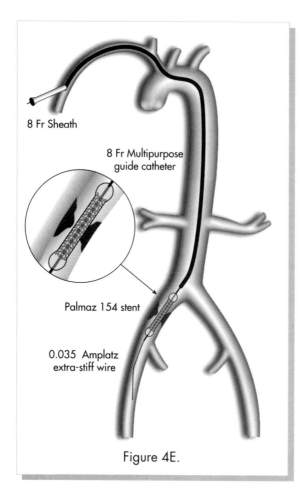

8 Fr Sheath

8 Fr Multipurpose guide catheter

Palmaz 154 stent

0.035 Amplatz extra-stiff wire

Figure 4E.

Figure 4E. Brachial access: Palmaz iliac artery stent deployment. Advance balloon-mounted to stent lesion within guiding catheter.

11.   Predilate the lesion.

a.   Inflate the balloon to the lowest pressure that results in complete balloon expansion. *(NB: If unable to completely expand the balloon, either abort stent attempt, or use a rotablator to release the constricting band of fibrous tissue or calcification and redilate)*

b.   Deflate the balloon and remove it, leaving the guidewire across the lesion.

12. Perform angiography through the guiding catheter to assess the results of balloon angioplasty.

13. Advance the guiding catheter across the lesion.

14. Hand-crimp an unmounted medium (4 mm to 9 mm diameter) Palmaz stent onto the predilation balloon, or use the crimping device supplied by the manufacture is used to mount the stent. *(NB: When*

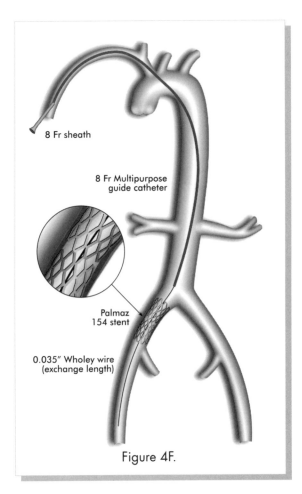

Figure 4F. Brachial access: Palmaz iliac artery stent deployment. Withdraw guiding catheter and deploy stent.

8 Fr sheath

8 Fr Multipurpose guide catheter

Palmaz 154 stent

0.035" Wholey wire (exchange length)

Figure 4F.

using the crimping device, remember to use the protective plastic sleeve to protect the stent.)

15. Advance the balloon-mounted stent to the level of the lesion within the guiding catheter. *(NB: By keeping the balloon-mounted stent within the guide catheter, the risk of stent embolism is minimized.)*

16. Withdraw the guiding catheter to "uncover" the stent at the lesion site. The placement of the stent is confirmed by reviewing the angiogram, performing contrast injections through the sheath, or by comparing the stent's relative position in the body to the previously selected landmarks.

17. Deploy the Palmaz stent with gradual inflation of the balloon so that a "dumb-bell" shape is created at both ends of the balloon. *(NB: This prevents asymmetric balloon inflation and avoids stent embolization or displacement during expansion.)* **(Figure 5 A)**

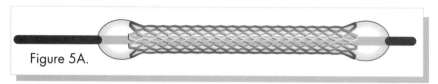

Figure 5A. Palmaz stent deployment. Gradual balloon inflation to form dumb-bell shape.

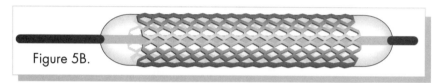

Figure 5B. Fully expand stent to 6 ATM.

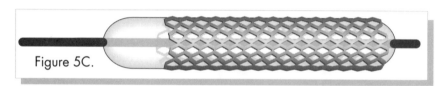

Figure 5C. Withdraw balloon so that distal margin is within stent and inflate to 8+ ATM.

18. Inflate the balloon to 6 ATM and deploy the stent. (**Figure 5 B**)

19. Withdraw the balloon, which is longer than the stent, so that the distal shoulder of the balloon is within the margins of the stent and inflate the balloon to higher pressures (8+ ATM) minimizing the risk of a dissection. (**Figure 5 C**)

20. Measure the pressure gradient across the stent through the balloon's wire lumen.

21. Remove the balloon, leaving the guidewire in place and perform angiography.

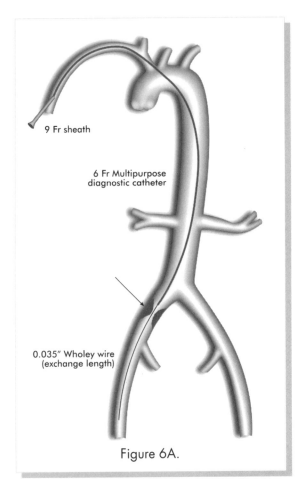

9 Fr sheath

6 Fr Multipurpose
diagnostic catheter

0.035" Wholey wire
(exchange length)

Figure 6A.

Figure 6A. Brachial
access: Wallstent deployment.
Insert 9 Fr sheath,
advance Wholey
wire across lesion.

VI. Wallstent iliac stent placement from brachial artery access (Figure 6 A - C)

1. Insert a 9 Fr (stent deployment with a guiding catheter) sheath either percutaneously or via cutdown into the brachial artery.

2. Administer 5,000 IU of heparin.

3. Direct a 0.035-in Wholey guidewire (exchange length) over the aortic arch to the descending aorta using either a 6 Fr pigtail or multipurpose catheter.

4. Exchange the diagnostic 6 Fr catheter for a 9 Fr multipurpose guiding catheter and place the wire and guiding catheter into the ostium

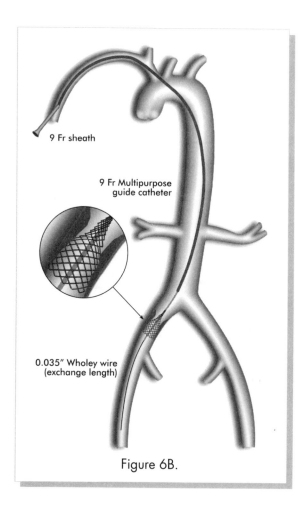

9 Fr sheath

9 Fr Multipurpose
guide catheter

0.035" Wholey wire
(exchange length)

Figure 6B.

Figure 6B. Brachial access: Wallstent deployment.

After predilation, advance Wallstent across lesion and begin deployment.

of the target iliac artery.

5.   Cross the iliac artery lesion with the steerable, atraumatic 0.035-in Wholey wire. (*NB: If the Wholey wire will not cross the lesion, a 0.035-in angled or straight Glidewire, or an 0.035-in straight extra-stiff Amplatz wire may be used.*)

6.   Using test injections of contrast, select the best view, either AP or an angled view, to demonstrate the lesion.

7.   Perform a baseline angiogram with the wire across the lesion.

8.   Measure the reference diameter of the vessel and the lesion length. (*NB: Visual estimation of vessels larger than 4.0 mm is quite variable and overdilation of an artery may lead to rupture or extensive dissection.*)

9.   Mark the location of the target lesion with bony landmarks, or with an external radiopaque ruler.

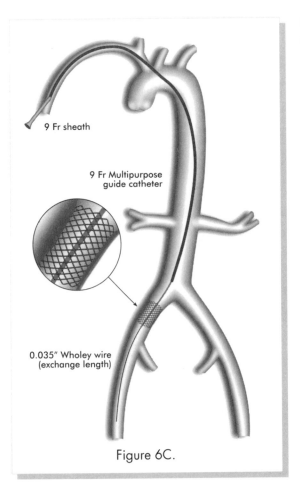

9 Fr sheath

9 Fr Multipurpose
guide catheter

0.035" Wholey wire
(exchange length)

Figure 6C.

Figure 6C. Brachial access: Wallstent deployment.
Complete deployment of Wallstent.

10. Advance a balloon catheter across the lesion, chosen to match the reference artery diameter (1:1), and long enough to cover the lesion.

a. Remove the Wholey wire and measure a hemodynamic gradient across the lesion, using the wire lumen of the balloon catheter and the guiding catheter/sheath.

b. Advance an exchange length Amplatz extra-stiff wire through the balloon wire lumen to the distal vessels to provide support for stent placement.

11. Predilate the lesion.

a. Inflate the balloon to the lowest pressure that results in complete balloon expansion. *(NB: If unable to completely expand the balloon, either abort stent attempt, or use a rotablator to release the constricting band of fibrous tissue or calcification and redilate)*

b. Deflate the balloon and remove it, leaving the guidewire across the lesion.

12. Perform angiography to assess the results of balloon angioplasty.

13. Select a self-expanding Wallstent to be at least 1 mm in diameter larger than the reference vessel diameter, and long enough to completely cover the lesion.

14. Advance the Wallstent through the guiding catheter, over the 0.035-in extra-stiff Amplatz wire and cross the lesion.

15. Guide the placement of the stent by either bony landmarks, an external ruler, or contrast injections through the guiding catheter.

16. Position the distal end of the Wallstent several centimeters distal to the distal margin of the target lesion.

17. Withdraw the constraining sheath about 1/4 of its length. *(NB: The Wallstent may be pulled back, but not advanced once the stent has begun to expand, so the operator should error on the side of distal placement, and make subsequent adjustments by withdrawal in small increments. It is possible to reconstrain the stent within the constraining sheath if the "point of no return" marked with a radiographic marker on the shaft of the delivery catheter has not been exceeded.)*

18. Completely withdraw the constraining sheath to fully deploy the stent.

19. Exchange the Wallstent delivery catheter for the predilation balloon catheter.

20. Inflate the balloon to 8+ ATM to ensure complete stent expansion, with the distal margin of the balloon within the stent. *(NB: This technique minimizes the risk of a distal dissection.)*

21. Measure the post-stent pressure gradient through the balloon lumen.

22. Remove the balloon and perform angiography.

VII. Palmaz iliac stent placement from ipsilateral (retrograde) femoral artery access (Figure 7 A - G)

1. Gain common femoral artery access with a 6 Fr sheath for medium (4 mm to 9 mm) or 8 Fr sheath for large (8 mm to 12 mm) Palmaz stent placement.
2. Administer 2,500 IU of heparin.
3. Cross the lesion with a steerable, atraumatic 0.035-in Wholey wire. *(NB: If the Wholey wire will not cross the lesion, a 0.035-in angled or straight Glidewire, or an 0.035-in straight extra-stiff Amplatz wire may be used.)*
4. Advance a 6 Fr pigtail catheter over the wire and across the lesion.
5. Remove the guidewire and measure a crossing gradient between the lumen of the pigtail catheter and the sheath.
6. Select the best view of the lesion with test injections.
7. Perform a baseline angiogram of the lesion.
8. Measure the reference diameter of the vessel and the lesion length. *(NB: Visual estimation of vessels larger than 4.0 mm is quite variable and overdilation of an artery may lead to rupture or extensive dissection.)*
9. Mark the location of the target lesion with bony landmarks, or with an external radiopaque ruler.
10. Advance an 0.035-in Amplatz extra-stiff wire to the aorta and remove the pigtail catheter.
11. Predilate the lesion with a balloon chosen to match the reference artery diameter, and long enough to cover the lesion.
12. The balloon is inflated to the lowest pressure that results in complete balloon expansion. *(NB: If unable to completely expand the balloon, either abort stent attempt, or use a rotablator to release the constricting band of fibrous tissue of calcification and redilate.)*
13. The balloon is deflated and removed, leaving the guidewire across the lesion.

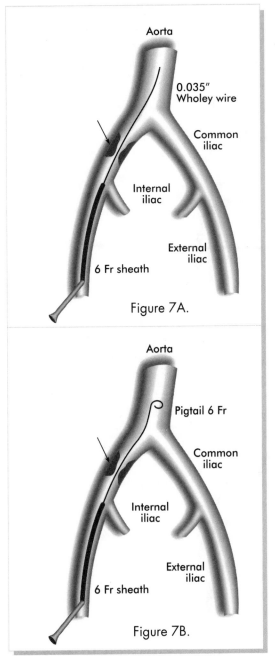

Figure 7A.

Figure 7B.

Figure 7A. Ipsilateral femoral access: Palmaz stent deployment.

6 Fr sheath in the common femoral artery, cross lesion with Wholey wire.

Figure 7B. Ipsilateral femoral access: Palmaz stent deployment.

Advance pigtail catheter across lesion to terminal aorta.

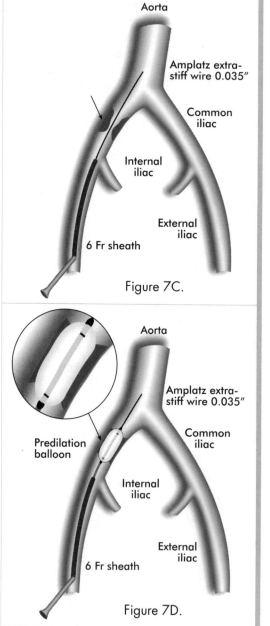

Figure 7C.

Figure 7D.

Figure 7C. Ipsilateral femoral access: Palmaz stent deployment.
Insert Amplatz extra-stiff wire and remove pigtail catheter.

Figure 7D. Ipsilateral femoral access: Palmaz stent deployment.
Predilate lesion.

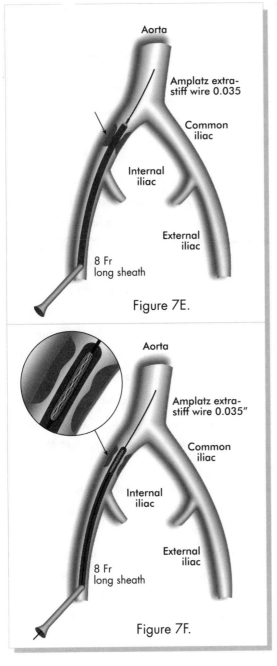

Figure 7E.

Figure 7F.

Figure 7E. Ipsilateral femoral access: Palmaz stent deployment.

Remove balloon, insert 8 Fr long sheath (P 308 stent) across lesion.

Figure 7F. Ipsilateral femoral access: Palmaz stent deployment.

Advance balloon-mounted P 308 stent within sheath to lesion site.

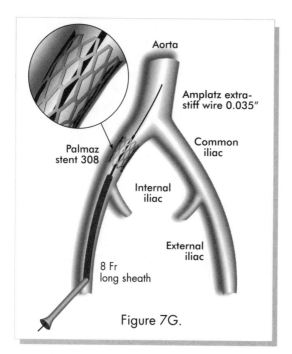

Aorta

Amplatz extra-
stiff wire 0.035"

Common
iliac

Palmaz
stent 308

Internal
iliac

External
iliac

8 Fr
long sheath

Figure 7G.

Figure 7G. Ipsilateral femoral access: Palmaz stent deployment.

Withdraw sheath to uncover stent and deploy stent to 6 ATM.

14. Perform angiography to assess the results of balloon angioplasty.

15. For a medium (4 mm to 9 mm diameter) Palmaz stent, a 6 Fr, 20 mm to 30 mm long sheath (long enough to cross the lesion. For large Palmaz stents (8 to 12+ mm expanded diameter) an 8 Fr, 20 mm to 30 mm long sheath is required.

16. Unmounted stents are hand-crimped onto the predilation balloon, or the crimping device supplied by the manufacture is used to mount the stent. *(NB: When using the crimping device, remember to use the plastic sleeve to protect the stent.)*

17. Insert the balloon-mounted stent through the diaphragm of sheath and advance it to the level of the lesion within the protected environment of the sheath.

18. Withdraw the sheath to "uncover" the stent at the lesion site. The placement of the stent is confirmed by reviewing the angiogram, performing contrast injections through the sheath, or by comparing the stent's relative position in the body to the previously selected landmarks.

19. Deploy the Palmaz stent with gradual inflation of the balloon so that a "dumb-bell" shape is created at both ends of the balloon. This prevents asymmetric balloon inflation and avoids stent embolization or displacement during expansion. *(NB: This prevents asymmetric balloon inflation and avoids stent embolization or displacement during expansion.)*

20. Inflate the balloon to 6 ATM and deploy the stent.

21. Withdraw the balloon, which is longer than the stent, so that the distal shoulder of the balloon is within the margins of the stent and inflate the balloon to higher pressures (8+ ATM) minimizing the risk of a dissection.

22. Measure the post-stent pressure gradient through the balloon lumen.

23. Remove the balloon, leaving the guidewire in place and perform angiography.

VIII. Wallstent iliac stent placement from ipsilateral (retrograde) femoral artery access (Figure 8 A)

1. Insert a 7 Fr sheath into the common femoral artery.

2. Administer 2,500 IU of heparin.

3. Cross the iliac artery lesion with the steerable, atraumatic 0.035-in Wholey wire. *(NB: If the Wholey wire will not cross the lesion, a 0.035-in angled or straight Glidewire, or an 0.035-in straight extra-stiff Amplatz wire may be used.)*

4. Advance a 6 Fr pigtail catheter over the wire and across the lesion.

5. Remove the guidewire and measure a crossing gradient between the lumen of the pigtail catheter and the sheath.

6. Select the best view of the lesion with test injections.

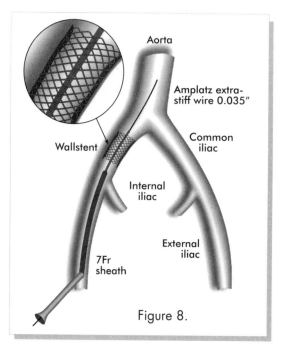

Aorta

Amplatz extra-stiff wire 0.035"

Wallstent

Common iliac

Internal iliac

External iliac

7Fr sheath

Figure 8.

Figure 8. Ipsilateral femoral access: Wallstent placement.

Using standard 7 Fr sheath, deploy Wallstent after predilation.

7.   Perform a baseline angiogram of the lesion.

8.   Measure the reference diameter of the vessel and the lesion length. *(NB: Visual estimation of vessels larger than 4.0 mm is quite variable and overdilation of an artery may lead to rupture or extensive dissection.)*

9. Mark the location of the target lesion with bony landmarks, or with an external radiopaque ruler.

10. Advance an 0.035-in Amplatz extra-stiff wire to the aorta and remove the pigtail catheter.

11. Predilate the lesion with a balloon chosen to match the reference artery diameter, and long enough to cover the lesion.

12. The balloon is inflated to the lowest pressure that results in complete balloon expansion. *(NB: If unable to completely expand the balloon, either abort stent attempt, or use a rotablator to release the constricting band of fibrous tissue or calcification and redilate.)*

13. The balloon is deflated and removed, leaving the guidewire across the lesion.

14. Perform angiography to assess the results of balloon angioplasty.

15. Select a self-expanding Wallstent to be at least 1 mm in diameter larger than the reference vessel diameter, and long enough to completely cover the lesion.

16. Advance the Wallstent through the guiding catheter/sheath, over the 0.035-in extra-stiff Amplatz wire and cross the lesion.

17. Guide the placement of the stent by either bony landmarks, an external ruler, or contrast injections through the arterial sheath or guiding catheter.

18. Position the Wallstent several centimeters beyond (distal) to the target lesion.

19. Withdraw the constraining sheath about 1/4 of its length. *(NB: The Wallstent may be pulled back, but not advanced once the stent has begun to expand, so the operator should err on the side of distal placement, and make subsequent adjustments by withdrawal in small increments. It is possible to reconstrain the stent within the constraining sheath if the "point of no return" marked with a radiographic marker on the shaft of the delivery catheter has not been exceeded.)*

20. Completely withdraw the constraining sheath to fully deploy the stent.

21. Exchange the Wallstent delivery catheter for the predilation balloon catheter.

22. Inflate the balloon to 8+ ATM, with the distal margin of the balloon within the stent, to ensure complete stent expansion.

23. Measure a final pressure gradient through the stent.

24. Remove the balloon and perform angiography.

IX. Palmaz iliac stent placement from contralateral femoral artery access (Figure 9 A - E)

1. Gain contralateral common femoral artery access with a 8 Fr sheath for medium (4 mm to 9 mm) Palmaz stent placement.
2. Administer 2,500 IU of heparin.
3. Advance a 6 Fr internal mammary artery (IMA) catheter over an exchange length 0.035-in angled Glidewire to the aorta.
4. Withdraw the IMA catheter to select the contralateral iliac artery.
5. Cross the lesion with the 0.035-in angled Glidewire.
6. Exchange the 6 Fr IMA catheter for an 8 Fr Crossover guiding catheter.
7. Select the best view of the lesion with test injections.
8. Perform a baseline angiogram of the lesion.
9. Measure the reference diameter of the vessel and the lesion length. *(NB: Visual estimation of vessels larger than 4.0 mm is quite variable and overdilation of an artery may lead to rupture or extensive dissection.)*
10. Mark the location of the target lesion with bony landmarks, or with an external radiopaque ruler.
11. Advance a balloon catheter across the lesion, chosen to match the reference artery diameter, and long enough to cover the lesion.
    a. Remove the Glidewire and measure a hemodynamic gradient across the lesion, using the wire lumen of the balloon catheter and the guiding catheter/sheath.
    b. Advance an exchange length 0.035-in Amplatz extra-stiff wire through the balloon wire lumen to the distal vessel.
12. Predilate the lesion.
    a. The balloon is inflated to the lowest pressure that results in complete balloon expansion. *(NB: If unable to completely expand the*

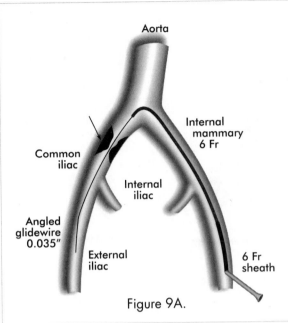

Figure 9A.

Aorta

Internal
mammary
6 Fr

Common
iliac

Internal
iliac

Angled
glidewire
0.035″

External
iliac

6 Fr
sheath

Figure 9A. Contralateral femoral access: Palmaz (medium 4 mm to 9 mm) stent deployment.

8 Fr sheath, 6 Fr internal mammary catheter and angled glidewire to gain contralateral iliac access.

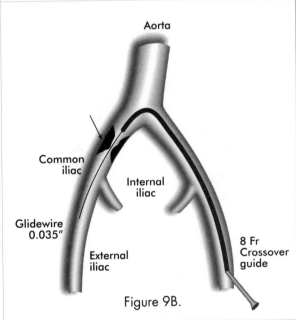

Figure 9B.

Aorta

Common
iliac

Internal
iliac

Glidewire
0.035″

External
iliac

8 Fr
Crossover
guide

Figure 9B. Contralateral femoral access: Palmaz (medium 4 mm to 9 mm) stent deployment.

Remove mammary catheter and place 8 Fr Crossover guide with predilation balloon. Exchange Glidewire for extra-stiff Amplatz wire after balloon is across the lesion.

CHAPTER TWO: ILIAC ARTERY

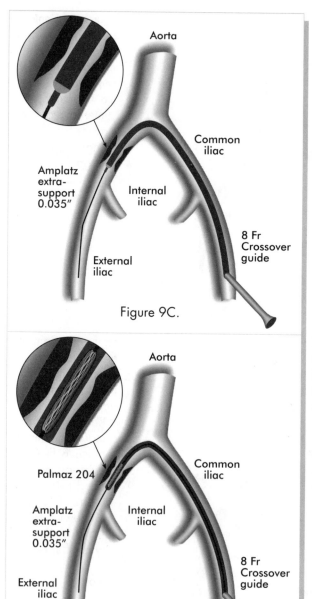

Aorta

Common
iliac

Amplatz
extra-
support
0.035″

Internal
iliac

8 Fr
Crossover
guide

External
iliac

Figure 9C.

Aorta

Palmaz 204

Common
iliac

Amplatz
extra-
support
0.035″

Internal
iliac

8 Fr
Crossover
guide

External
iliac

Figure 9D.

Figure 9C. Con-
tralateral femoral ac-
cess: Palmaz (me-
dium 4 mm to 9 mm)
stent deployment.
Advance Cross-
over guide across
lesion after predi-
lation.

Figure 9D. Contralat-
eral femoral access:
Palmaz (medium 4
mm to 9 mm) stent
deployment.
Advance balloon-
mounted stent to
lesion site within
the Crossover
guide.

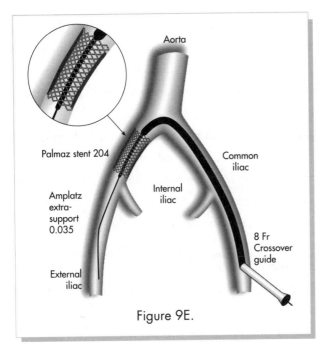

Aorta

Palmaz stent 204

Common iliac

Internal iliac

Amplatz extra-support 0.035

8 Fr Crossover guide

External iliac

Figure 9E.

balloon, either abort stent attempt, or use a rotablator to release the constricting band of fibrous tissue or calcification and redilate.)

b. The balloon is deflated and removed, leaving the Amplatz extra-stiff wire across the lesion.

13. Perform angiography to assess the results of balloon angioplasty.

14. Advance the Crossover guiding catheter across the lesion.

15. Hand-crimp an unmounted medium (4 mm to 9 mm diameter) Palmaz stent onto the predilation balloon, or use the crimping device supplied by the manufacture is used to mount the stent. (NB: When using the crimping device, remember to use the protective plastic sleeve to protect the stent.)

16. Advance the balloon-mounted stent to the level of the lesion within the guiding catheter.

17. Withdraw the guiding catheter to "uncover" the stent at the lesion site. The placement of the stent is confirmed by reviewing the angiogram, performing contrast injections through the guide catheter, or by comparing the stent's relative position in the body to the previously selected landmarks.

18. Deploy the Palmaz stent with gradual inflation of the balloon so that a "dumb-bell" shape is created at both ends of the balloon. *(NB: This prevents asymmetric balloon inflation and avoids stent embolization or displacement during expansion.)*

19. Inflate the balloon to 6 ATM and deploy the stent.

20. Withdraw the balloon, which is longer than the stent, so that the distal shoulder of the balloon is within the margins of the stent and inflate the balloon to higher pressures (8+ ATM) minimizing the risk of a dissection.

21. Measure a final gradient through the balloon wire lumen.

22. Remove the balloon, leaving the guidewire in place and perform angiography.

X. Wallstent iliac stent placement from contralateral femoral artery access (Figure 10 A & B)

1. Gain contralateral common femoral artery access with a 7 Fr sheath.

2. Administer 2,500 IU of heparin.

3. Advance a 6 Fr internal mammary artery (IMA) catheter over an exchange length 0.035-in angled Glidewire to the aorta.

4. Withdraw the IMA catheter to select the contralateral iliac artery.

5. Cross the lesion with the 0.035-in angled Glidewire.

6. Exchange the 6 Fr IMA catheter for a 7 Fr Crossover sheath catheter.

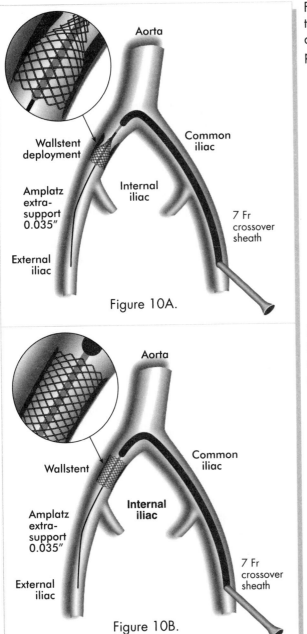

Figure 10A.

Figure 10B.

Labels in Figure 10A:
Aorta
Common iliac
Wallstent deployment
Internal iliac
Amplatz extra-support 0.035"
7 Fr crossover sheath
External iliac

Labels in Figure 10B:
Aorta
Common iliac
Wallstent
Internal iliac
Amplatz extra-support 0.035"
7 Fr crossover sheath
External iliac

Figure 10A. Contralateral femoral access: Wallstent placement.

Using a 7 Fr. Crossover sheath, advance the Wallstent across the lesion following predilation.

41

Figure 10B. Contralateral femoral access: Wallstent placement.

Complete deployment of Wallstent.

7. Select the best view of the lesion with test injections.

8. Perform a baseline angiogram of the lesion.

9. Measure the reference diameter of the vessel and the lesion length. *(NB: Visual estimation of vessels larger than 4.0 mm is quite variable and overdilation of an artery may lead to rupture or extensive dissection.)*

10. Mark the location of the target lesion with bony landmarks, or with an external radiopaque ruler.

11. Advance a balloon catheter across the lesion, chosen to match the reference artery diameter, and long enough to cover the lesion.

    a. Remove the Glidewire and measure a hemodynamic gradient across the lesion, using the wire lumen of the balloon catheter and the guiding catheter/sheath.

    b. Advance an exchange length 0.035-in Amplatz extra-stiff wire through the balloon wire lumen to the distal vessel.

12. Predilate the lesion.

    a. The balloon is inflated to the lowest pressure that results in complete balloon expansion. *(NB: If unable to completely expand the balloon, either abort stent attempt, or use a rotablator to release the constricting band of fibrous tissue or calcification and redilate.)*

    b. The balloon is deflated and removed, leaving the Amplatz extra-stiff wire across the lesion.

13. Perform angiography to assess the results of balloon angioplasty.

14. Select a self-expanding Wallstent to be at least 1 mm in diameter larger than the reference vessel diameter, and long enough to completely cover the lesion.

15. Advance the Wallstent through the guiding catheter, over the 0.035-in extra-stiff Amplatz wire and cross the lesion.

16. Guide the placement of the stent by either bony landmarks, an external ruler, or contrast injections through the guiding catheter.

17. Position the Wallstent several centimeters distal to the target lesion.

18. Withdraw the constraining sheath about 1/4 of its length. *(NB: The Wallstent may be pulled back, but not advanced once the stent has begun to expand, so the operator should err on the side of distal placement, and make subsequent adjustments by withdrawal in small increments. It is possible to reconstrain the stent within the constraining sheath if the "point of no return" marked with a radiographic marker on the shaft of the delivery catheter has not been exceeded.)*

19. Completely withdraw the constraining sheath to fully deploy the stent.

20. Exchange the Wallstent delivery catheter for the balloon catheter.

21. Inflate the balloon to 8+ ATM, with the distal margin of the balloon within the stent, to ensure complete stent expansion.

22. Measure the post-stent pressure gradient through the balloon lumen.

23. Remove the balloon and perform final angiography.

XI. Assessing the results of stent placement

1. Angiography.

   a. Assess stent expansion relative to the reference diameter.

      1) Generally, there should be a slight over-expansion of the stent to produce a "step-up and step-down" effect.

      2) If a significant ($\geq 20\%$) diameter stenosis remains, the stent should be dilated either with a larger balloon or at higher pressure using the original balloon. *(NB: Remember that compliant balloons will enlarge significantly at higher pressures.)*

   b. Determine that there is good distal run-off, and no proximal or distal dissection of vessel has occurred which could impair either inflow or outflow from the treated lesion.

      1) If run-off is sluggish, search proximally and distally for its cause. Poor flow will jeopardize stent patency.

2) If a flow-limiting dissection is discovered it should be treated with additional balloon inflations or a second stent.

2. Measure the final translesional hemodynamic gradient

   a. The final translesional gradient may be measured with the post-dilation balloon or with an angiographic catheter across lesion.

   b. The gradient across the lesion should be resolved with stent placement. It is acceptable to terminate the procedure, however, once the gradient has been reduced to less than 5 mmHg.

3. Perform intravascular ultrasound (IVUS) imaging (optional). *(NB: Most IVUS systems will require that you exchange the 0.035-in wire for a 0.014-in guidewire.)*

   a. The stent minimal lumen diameter (MLD) should be equal to or slightly larger than the reference vessel MLD. *(NB: Care must be taken not to overdilate stents in long segments of tapering arteries.)*

   b. The stent struts should be circumferentially apposed to vessel wall. If non-apposition of stent struts is identified, redilation with larger balloons or at higher pressures is recommended. *(NB: Remember that compliant balloons will enlarge significantly at higher pressures.)*

   c. The inflow and outflow portion of the stented segment should be carefully checked for dissection. Large dissections, or flow limiting dissections require treatment with additional balloon inflations or additional stents.

XII. Sheath removal and post-procedure care

1. Remove the sheath when the ACT is ≤ 170 seconds.

2. Ipsilateral retrograde femoral access: Care should be taken when removing the femoral sheath after ipsilateral stent placement.

Overcompression of the femoral artery may lead to stasis of flow and stent thrombosis. The goal is to apply enough pressure to tamponade bleeding without causing femoral artery occlusion. Another option is to use one of the several vessel closure devices, which avoids prolonged compression of the vessel.

3. Discharge the patient on daily aspirin when stable, usually within 24 hours of the stent procedure.

4. Measure the post treatment ankle-brachial index (ABI) prior to discharge to establish a new baseline for future comparison.

XIII. Lesion specific techniques

1. Acute iliac occlusions: Iliac occlusion is an accepted indication for stent placement due to the generally poor results and the increased restenosis rate after PTA alone. Acute thrombosis of an iliac artery can be a limb-threatening emergency. Access is gained away from the "culprit" lesion, either from the brachial approach or the contralateral femoral artery. (**Figure 11 A - E**).

   a. Emergency diagnostic infrarenal abdominal angiography with run-off is performed to delineate the culprit lesion, and to assess the inflow and outflow vessels.

   b. The iliac occlusion is crossed with a guidewire. The atraumatic 0.035-in Wholey wire should be tried first, but if this fails, use an angled or straight Glidewire to cross the lesion.

   c. If an extensive clot burden is present, urokinase infused at 1,000 units to 4,000 units per minute (60 thousand to 240 thousand units per hour) or rtPA at 0.05 mg/kg/hr may be administered. After a 4 hour infusion, the lesion is rechecked and if lysis has been successful, definitive therapy with stent placement can proceed.

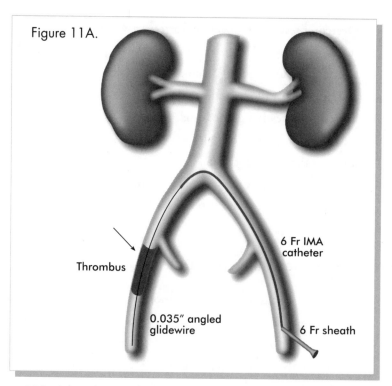

Figure 11A.

Thrombus

6 Fr IMA catheter

0.035" angled glidewire

6 Fr sheath

Figure 11A. Acute iliac occlusion: Recanalization.
6 Fr sheath and contralateral femoral access, 6 Fr internal mammary artery catheter and cross thrombus with Glidewire.

  d. For discrete lesions with minimal thrombus burden, we perform direct angioplasty and stent placement.

2. Chronic iliac occlusions: Chronic occlusions (≥ 1 month old) of the iliac artery are generally approached in a retrograde fashion from the ipsilateral femoral artery. The advantage of the retrograde approach is that the guidewire does not have to negotiate side-branches, which may cause difficulty when crossing the lesion in an antegrade manner.

  a. Obtain ipsilateral (retrograde) femoral access with a 6 Fr sheath and administer 2,500 IU to 5,000 IU of heparin.

  b. Cross the lesion with an angled or straight Glidewire. If this

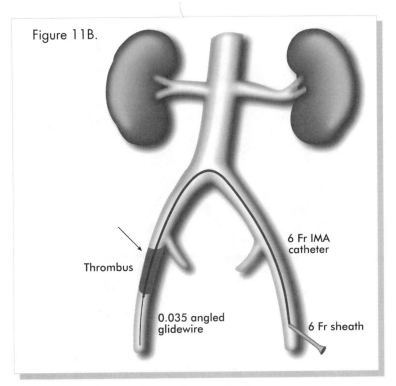

Figure 11B.

Thrombus

6 Fr IMA
catheter

0.035 angled
glidewire

6 Fr sheath

Figure 11B. Acute iliac occlusion: Recanalization.
Advance 6 Fr internal mammary catheter across thrombus.

fails, an 0.035-in extra-stiff Amplatz wire may be tried. We have found that the soft Wholey wire is rarely successful in crossing chronic total occlusions.

c. Perform diagnostic angiography with a 6 Fr pigtail catheter across the lesion and placed in the infra-renal abdominal aorta to image the lesion, as well as its inflow and outflow vessels. It is critical to note any collateral circulation that has developed to the affected leg.

d. Place an extra-stiff, 0.035-in Amplatz wire through the 6 Fr pigtail into the abdominal aorta and remove the diagnostic catheter leaving the wire in place.

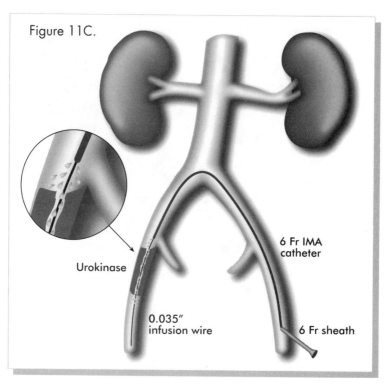

Figure 11C. Acute iliac occlusion: Recanalization.
Inject 250 kU of urokinase as the catheter is withdrawn through the thrombus (lacing). Begin local arterial infusion of urokinase.

  e. Perform iliac angioplasty and stent placement over the extra-stiff Amplatz guidewire.

3. Lengthy iliac occlusions: Lengthy (≥ 6 cm) chronic occlusions or those that appear to contain significant thrombus may be candidates for selective thrombolysis prior to angioplasty and stent placement. Thrombolysis often transforms long occlusions into much more discrete lesions.

  a. Gain access from the contralateral femoral artery if possible which minimizes bleeding complications that may occur when infusing

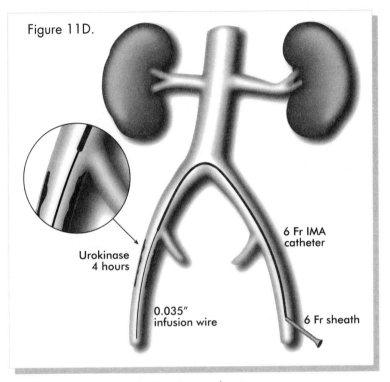

Figure 11D.

Urokinase
4 hours

6 Fr IMA
catheter

0.035"
infusion wire

6 Fr sheath

Figure 11D. Acute iliac occlusion: Recanalization.
Angiographic re-look at 4 hours after infusion of UK.

lytic agents immediatly proximal to the access site. Admininster 2,500 IU to 5,000 IU of heparin.

b. If the lesion can be crossed with a wire, a multi-holed infusion catheter is placed across the lesion. If the lesion cannot be crossed with a wire, an end-hole catheter is placed against the occlusion and the infusion started. Urokinase should be infused at 1,000 units to 4,000 units per minute (60 thousand to 240 thousand units per hour). The patient should be systemically anticoagulated with heparin to maintain the APTT between 60 sec and 80 sec.

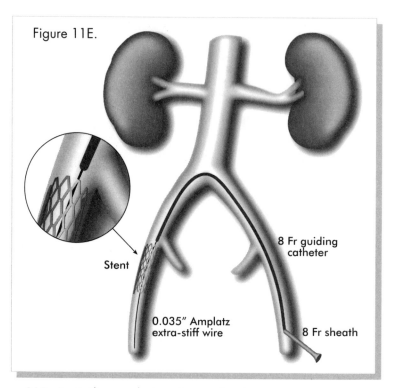

Figure 11E.

Stent

8 Fr guiding catheter

0.035" Amplatz extra-stiff wire

8 Fr sheath

Figure 11E. Acute iliac occlusion: Recanalization.
Insert 8 Fr Crossover guiding catheter and deploy stent.

c. After 4 to 6 hours, the lesion is rechecked to determine whether to continue the infusion.

d. If there has been little or no improvement at 4 to 6 hours, we abandon the lytic infusion and attempt to treat the lesion with direct angioplasty and stent placement.

e. If progress has occurred, the infusion may be continued and the dose adjusted to maximize the beneficial effect, which generally results in a more discrete and favorable lesion for treatment.

4. Aorto-iliac bifurcation: Aorto-iliac bifurcation lesions are approached with bilateral retrograde femoral artery access.

a. Each lesion is crossed with a guidewire and angiography is performed.

b. Predilation is performed with simutaneous inflation of two balloons, sized for each iliac artery. Long (30 cm) femoral sheaths are advanced across the lesions.

c. Palmaz stents (either medium or large) are mounted on the balloons used for predilation, and positioned several millimeters above the iliac bifurcation. The stents are deployed with simultaneous balloon inflation, resulting in the formation of a new iliac bifurcation.

5. Internal iliac involvement: Iliac lesions involving the internal iliac artery pose a problem of placing the internal iliac in "stent jail", and the increased risk of sidebranch vessel closure during stent deployment.

a. If the ostium of the internal iliac artery is involved in the common iliac artery lesion it can be dilated and stented from the contralateral approach before a stent is placed in the common iliac artery.

b. If the internal iliac artery is small, or the contralateral internal iliac artery is patent, then the common iliac artery may be treated, and the potential risk of sidebranch closure (10% to 15%) can be accepted.

c. If the involved internal iliac provides critical collateral flow, then its patency needs to be assured, or the common iliac artery lesion treated with surgery.

6. External iliac artery lesions have a propensity for dissection with balloon dilation alone. Care must be taken as the lesion potentially involves the common femoral artery (hip joint) and require flexible stents. Also, if a stent is placed in the common femoral artery, that access site for percutaneous procedures is lost.

XIV. Troubleshooting

1. **Tortuosity:** Severe vessel tortuosity can make iliac stent deployment difficult.

   a. Wire position across the lesion should be gained with a flexible, steerable wire.

   b. A flexible small diameter catheter (4 Fr multipurpose) is advanced across the lesion and the flexible wire may then be exchanged for a stiffer wire, which will help to straighten the tortuous vessel.

   c. The stent delivery sheath may then be advanced over the stiffer guidewire.

2. **Recrossing stents:** Recrossing deployed stents in the iliac arteries is generally not technically difficult.

   a. All deployed stents should be recrossed with "J" tipped guidewire to avoid passing the wire through the stent struts or between the stent and vessel wall. **(Figure 12)**.

   b. When placing a second Palmaz stent through a stent, the sheath and dilator are re-advanced across the deployed stent to avoid having the stent struts of the second stent catch on first stent. *(NB: Avoid attempting to cross a deployed stent with a "bare" Palmaz stent.)*

3. **Stent embolization and retrieval:**

   a. If the stent is pushed backwards off of the balloon and onto the shaft of the balloon catheter, the balloon should be withdrawn, the stent will meet resistance at the sheath diaphragm and can be re-mounted by pulling the balloon into the stent.

   b. If the unexpanded stent is pushed off the front of the balloon and onto guidewire, care must be taken not withdraw the guidewire.

      1) Attempts to remount the stent onto a new "lower profile"

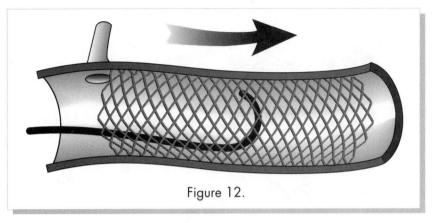

Figure 12.

Figure 12. Recrossing stents with a "J" wire.

balloon may be carefully tried. Again, care should be taken not to push the stent off of the guidewire. Once remounted, the stent may be repositioned at the lesion site and deployed. If this proves difficult, the stent may be deployed at a non-obstructive location in the artery, and the lesion treated with a second stent.

2) If attempts to remount the embolized stent fails, the undeployed stent may be retrieved with a loop snare and pulled back into the delivery sheath for removal. (**Figure 13**) The loop snare is placed over the guidewire and advanced to the stent (which is still on the wire). The rearmost portion of the stent is secured in the snare, and the stent, and the guidewire are withdrawn as a single unit under fluoroscopic visualization to the femoral sheath. Once the stent is within the sheath, the sheath is removed with the stent inside. The guidewire must remain in place to preserve vascular access.

c. If the stent is expanded or partially expanded and embolizes off

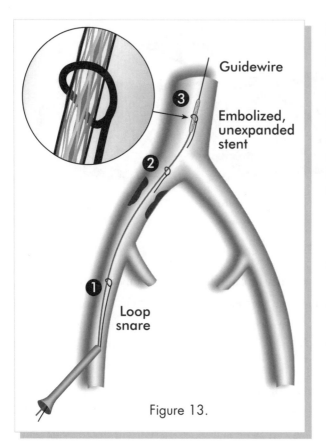

Guidewire

Embolized,
unexpanded
stent

Loop
snare

Figure 13.

Figure 13. With the embolized stent on the guidewire, advance the loop snare over the guidewire to the stent. Engage the stent and tighten the snare. Remove the stent and guidewire.

of the front of the balloon it will not be able to be retrieved through the sheath.

1) The balloon may be reformatted to lower its profile or a new balloon may be reinserted into the stent and the stent fully deployed at a non-obstructive location.

2) A more complicated technique involves using the loop snare to "recrimp" the stent to a diameter that will allow sheath extraction. The loop snare is advanced over the partially

deployed stent and tightened on the deployed stent to narrow its diameter. This is done multiple times to narrow the stent so that it will fit into a sheath. Occasionally, it is necessary to insert a larger sheath (14 Fr or 18 Fr) to facilitate stent removal. *(NB: Manipulation of partially deployed stents and retrieval of stents in a diseased aorta or iliac artery can easily damage the vessel or result in distal embolization of atherosclerotic debris.)*

4. **Dissection:** Dissection distal or proximal to stent should be assessed for severity. If minor, no treatment is necessary. However, the placement of a second stent is often indicated to ensure stent patency. The procedure for placing a second Palmaz stent involves recrossing the deployed stent with the dilator/sheath to insure passage of the stent through the deployed stent. The stents should be overlapped a minimal amount.

ILIAC STENT EQUIPMENT

Name	Company	Size	Length
Arterial/Venous Percutaneous Catheter Introducer Set			
Brite–tip	Cordis	6,7,8,9 Fr	11,23,35,45,55,90 cm
Flex	USCI	6,7,8,9 Fr	11,23 cm
Daig	Daig	5.5,7.5 Fr	90 cm
Pinnacle	Medi–tech	5–11 Fr	10,25 cm
Balkin Flexor Check–Flo	Cook	5.5,6,7,8 Fr	40 cm
Balkin Performer Check–Flo	Cook	5.5,6,7,8 Fr	40 cm
Angiography Catheters			
Pigtail, Multipurpose, IMA, Cobra, others	Various	6 Fr	~ 40–125 cm
Interventional Guiding Catheters			
Crossover, Hockey Stick, Multipurpose, others	Various	6–9 Fr	~ 45–90 cm
Guidewires			
J–wire, Amplatz extra–stiff, Bentson (soft)	Various	.035 in	~145–260 cm
Wholey	Mallinckrodt	.035 in	145,260 cm
Glide, angle (reg/stiff)	Medi–tech	.035 in	180,260 cm
Glide, straight (stiff)	Medi–tech	.035 in	260 cm
Roadrunner extra–support	Cook	.018 in	180,270,300 cm
Storq	Cordis	.035,.038 in	180,300 cm
PTA Dilatation Catheters			
Marshal	Medi–tech	4–10 mm x 1.5,2,3,4,6,8 cm	75,90,135 cm
Blue–Max	Medi–tech	4–12 mm x 2,3,4,8,10 cm	40,75,100,120 cm
XXL	Medi–tech	12–18 mm x 2,4,6 cm	75,120 cm

ILIAC STENT EQUIPMENT

Name	Company	Size	Length
Ultra–Thin Diamond	Medi–tech	4–10 mm x 1.5,2,3,4,6,8,10 cm	40,75,120,135 cm
Opta LP	Cordis	4–12 mm x 2,4,6,8,10 cm	65,80,110,135 cm
Powerflex plus	Cordis	4–12 mm x 2,4,6,8,10 cm	65,80,110,135 cm
Extreme	Cordis	4–10 mm x 2,4,6 cm	65,80,120 cm
Maxi	Cordis	14–20 mm x 2,4,6,8 cm	65,80,120 cm
Pursuit	Cook	4–10 mm	80,120 cm
Accent	Cook	4–12 mm	40,80,100,120 cm
Stents			
Palmaz medium	Cordis	4–9 mm	10,15,20,29,39 mm
Palmaz large	Cordis	8–12 mm	8,18,30 mm
Palmaz XL	Cordis	10–25 mm	30,40,50 mm
Palmaz Corinthian	Cordis	4–9 mm	60,80,100 mm
Corinthian IQ	Cordis	4–9 mm	12,15,18,29,39 mm
Smart	Cordis	6–14 mm	20,40,60,80 mm
Wallstent RP	Medi–tech	5–16 mm	20,40,60,90 mm
Wallstent (large)	Medi–tech	16–24 mm	35,45,70 mm
Bridge Flexible Biliary Plus	Medtronic AVE	6–10 mm	28,40,60,80,100 mm
Thrombolysis Systems			
EDM	Mallinckrodt	6,9,15 cm	145 cm
Tracker	Target	.018,.025,.038 in	150 cm
Mewissen	Medi–tech	5 Fr/5,10 cm	35,65,100 cm
Katzen	Medi–tech	3,6,9,12 cm	145,180 cm
Ultra–Fuse	Scimed	4,8 cm	140 cm
Transit	Cordis	3 Fr	85,100,135,150,170 cm
Mass Transit	Cordis	3 Fr	105,135 cm
Roubin	Cook	2.5–4 Fr	140 cm
Retrieval Systems			
Snare	Microvena	2,5,10,15 mm loop	120 cm
Dotter	Cook	3 cm diameter, 7 cm length	95 cm

57

Chapter Three

RENAL ARTERY STENT PLACEMENT

RENAL ARTERY STENT PLACEMENT

I. Indications for renal artery stent placement (Table 1)

1. Following a suboptimal angioplasty result in patients with renal artery stenosis associated with poorly controlled hypertension and/or renal insufficiency.
2. Lesions not suitable for balloon angioplasty.
   a. Aorto-ostial lesions (atherosclerotic).
   b. Restenotic lesions.

II. Diagnosis of renovascular hypertension (Table 2)

1. Patients at increased risk for renovascular hypertension include:
   a. New onset of hypertension < 30 yrs or > 55 yrs.
   b. Hypertension resistant to three drug medical therapy.
   c. Deterioration of renal function with ACE inhibitor therapy.
   d. Malignant hypertension.
   e. Abdominal or flank bruit.
   f. Associated atherosclerotic disease.
2. Screening tests for renovascular hypertension.

Table 1. Renovascular Hypertension: Prevalence

Clinical Population	Incidence (%)
All hypertensive patients	0.4
Hypertension and suspected coronary disease	20
Hypertension and peripheral vascular disease	30
Accelerated hypertension	40

a. Contrast aortography is the diagnostic procedure of choice in patients in whom the suspicion of renovascular hypertension is increased.

) In patients undergoing cardiac catheterization for suspected coronary disease with poorly controlled hypertension on two or more medications we routinely perform contrast aortog-

Table 2. Clinical Suspicion of Renovascular Hypertension

Hypertension onset < 30 yrs or > 55 yrs	Atrophic kidney or discrepant size of kidneys
Prior stable hypertension, now uncontrolled	Azotemia with ACE inhibitors
Malignant or accelerated hypertension	Azotemia in elderly with known atherosclerosis
Resistant hypertension	Abdominal/flank bruit (systolic and diastolic)

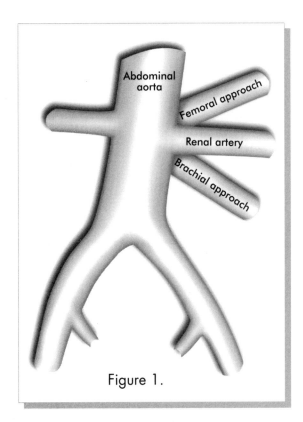

Figure 1.

Figure 1. Diagram of variable angulation of renal artery from aorta which may favor an arterial access site for stent placement.

raphy to visualize the renal arteries.

2)   In patients with renal failure, selective renal artery injections with as little as 3 cc of contrast will sufficiently opacify the renal artery to make a diagnosis of renal artery stenosis.

b.   Renal   vein renins: lateralizing renal vein renins have a high predictive value for improvement in blood pressure after treatment, but non-lateralizing renins have a low predictive accuracy for diagnosis and should not be relied upon to rule-out renovascular hypertension.

c.   Captopril renography: In our experience captopril renography is an expensive, time-consuming test with inadequate sensitivity to rule-out renal artery stenosis in patients at increased risk. It may be useful in patients who are unwilling to undergo contrast aortography.

d.   Spiral CT with contrast: This test requires the administration of radiographic contrast. Its usefulness as a screening test for renal artery stenosis is unknown.

e. Magnetic resonance angiography: This test does not require radiographic contrast. Its accuracy for detecting renal artery stenosis is compromised by the occurrence of "drop-out" artifacts where turbulent flow occurs, particularly at the ostia of the renal arteries.

f. Duplex imaging: Doppler and ultrasound imaging have a high specificity and very good sensitivity when performed by a skilled technician.

III. Performing diagnostic renal angiography

1. Choosing a vascular access site (**Figure 1**).

a. Brachial artery access: This site is preferred if intervention is planned when the renal arteries are oriented cranially.

1) Obtain access either percutaneously or by cutdown and insert a 6 Fr sheath.

2) Administer 5,000 IU of heparin.

3) Advance an 0.035-in J-guidewire to the aorta (descending aorta).

4) Advance a 6 Fr pigtail catheter over the wire to the aortic arch.

5) Use the pigtail catheter to direct the guidewire over the aortic arch to the descending aorta. It may be necessary to use a steerable wire such as a glidewire (Terumo) or Wholey wire to select the descending aorta.

6) Advance the pigtail catheter to the level of the renal arteries (L1 - L2) in preparation for angiography. Perform a test injection.

b. Femoral artery access: This site is preferred if intervention is planned when the renal arteries are oriented caudally or horizontally.

1) Insert a 6 Fr sheath retrogradely into the common femoral artery.

2) Administer 3,000 IU of heparin.

3) Advance an 0.035-in J-guidewire to the abdominal aorta.

4) Advance a 6 Fr pigtail catheter to the level of the renal arteries (L1 - L2). Perform a test injection.

2. Performing the diagnostic renal aortogram

a. Position the 6 Fr pigtail catheter so that the sideholes of the catheter are at the level of renal arteries, confirmed with test injections of contrast. *(NB: Placement of the catheter at too high a level will fill the superior mesenteric artery (SMA) which may obscure the ostium of the right renal artery.)*

b. Perform cineangiography with a 9-inch image intensifier at 12.5 frames/sec to 15 frames/sec in the anterior-posterior (AP) or 5 degree LAO projection. We prefer to use a low osmolar, low viscosity, ionic contrast (Hexabrix-320) or non-ionic contrast. The injection rate, using a power injector, is from 15 cc to 20 cc per second for 2 or 3 seconds. It is important to visualize accessory renal arteries if they are present. *(NB: Subtraction angiography of the aorta and renal arteries may be performed to conserve contrast, but limits the operator's ability to pan the distal aorta and common iliac arteries during the contrast injection. Generally, high quality subtraction images can be obtained with 20 to 30 cc of contrast injected over 2 seconds.)*

3. Perform selective renal angiography

a Selective renal angiography from the brachial approach is performed with a 6 Fr multipurpose catheter and hand injections of contrast.

b. Selective renal angiography from the femoral approach is performed with either a 6 Fr Judkins right coronary catheter, an internal mammary artery catheter, or a Cobra shaped catheter. Occasionally, a "shepherd's crook" catheter such as Simmon's I, II, or III catheters may be useful.

1) Hand injections of contrast are used to fill the renal artery, taking care to "reflux" contrast into the aorta to visualize the ostial portion of the vessel.

2) Care should be taken to avoid "scraping" catheters along the aortic wall when locating the renal artery arteries due to the risk of causing atheroemboli.

c. Optimal angiographic views are either antero-posterior (A-P) or slightly angled (5° LAO) to best define the lesion.

IV. Preparation for renal artery stent placement

1. Premedicate the patient with 325 mg of aspirin daily.

2. Anticoagulate the patient during the procedure with 3,000 IU to 5,000 IU of heparin.

3. Palmaz medium (biliary) stent delivery catheters will vary depending on the choice of vascular access.

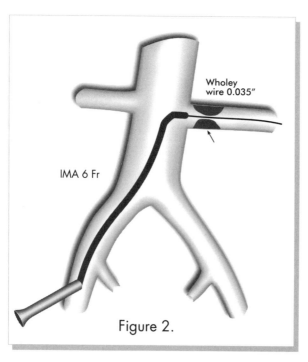

IMA 6 Fr

Wholey wire 0.035"

Figure 2.

Figure 2. Engage the renal artery with a diagnostic 6 Fr catheter and advance an exchange length 0.035-in Wholey wire across the lesion.

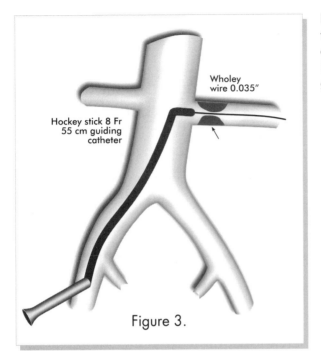

Figure 3. Exchange the diagnostic catheter for an 8 Fr Hockey stick (55 cm) guide catheter.

Wholey wire 0.035"

Hockey stick 8 Fr 55 cm guiding catheter

Figure 3.

a. From the brachial approach, an 8 Fr coronary guiding catheter (multipurpose) or a long (90cm) 6 Fr sheath is required to deliver a medium-sized Palmaz stent.

b. From the femoral approach an 8 Fr guiding catheter is required. We prefer to use a short (55 cm) Hockey stick or Renal (short, normal, or long-tip) guiding catheter.

V. Technique for renal stent placement

1. Gain vascular access at the selected site and administer 3,000 to 5,000 IU of heparin.

2. Engage the renal ostium with a diagnostic 6 Fr catheter.

3. Cross the lesion with a exchange length Wholey 0.035-in steerable wire (**Figure 2**). *(NB: Avoid using the Glidewire to cross renal lesions due to the risk of dissection and inadvertant distal perforation.)*

4. Exchange the diagnostic catheter for a guiding catheter or sheath (**Figure 3**).

5. Perform a baseline angiogram in the best working view with the guidewire across the lesion. *(NB: The guidewire across the lesion may significantly alter the orientation of the renal artery from its appearance on the diagnostic aortogram.)*

   a. For aorto-ostial lesions it is important that this view shows the origin of the renal vessel to guide stent placement.

   b. It is also important at this time to note any bony landmarks that will help to guide stent placement.

6. Perform on-line quantitative measurements to determine the reference vessel diameter. *(NB: Visual estimation of vessels larger than 4.0 mm is quite variable and overdilation of a renal artery may lead to rupture or extensive distal dissection.)*

7. Advance the predilation balloon (sized 1:1 with the reference vessel diameter) across the lesion (**Figure 4**). A baseline pressure gradient may be measured at this time through the guidewire lumen of the balloon.

8. Inflate the balloon to achieve complete expansion. Be aware that compliant balloons will enlarge at higher pressures. *(NB: If unable to completely expand the balloon, either abort stent attempt, or use a rotablator to release the constricting band of fibrous tissue or calcification and redilate.)*

9. Withdraw the balloon and perform an angiogram to assess balloon angioplasty result.

10. Readvance balloon across the lesion and insert the guiding catheter/sheath into the renal artery over the balloon across the lesion (**Figure 5**). *(NB: This technique helps to minimize the risk of stent embolization.)*

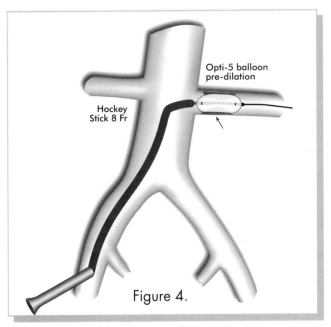

Figure 4.

Figure 4. Advance the predilation balloon across the lesion.

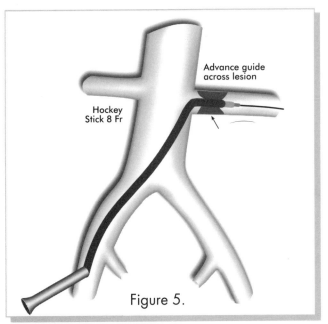

Figure 5.

Figure 5. Deflate the balloon and advance the guiding catheter over the balloon and across the lesion.

CHAPTER THREE: RENAL ARTERY

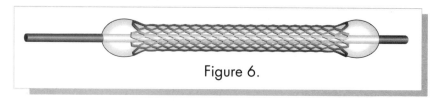

Figure 6.

Figure 6. Gradually inflate the balloon to 3 ATM to create a dumb-bell shape.

11. Remove the balloon leaving the wire and guide catheter/sheath across the lesion.

12. Select a Palmaz medium stent to cover lesion (10, 15 or 20 mm length). *(NB: We prefer to work with non-articulated stents to provide better lesion coverage with the stent.)*

13. Hand crimp the stent on the pre-dilation balloon.

14. Advance the stent mounted on the balloon within guide catheter/sheath to the lesion site.

15. Withdraw the guide catheter/sheath to uncover stent at the lesion site.

16. Using contrast injections from the guiding catheter posi-

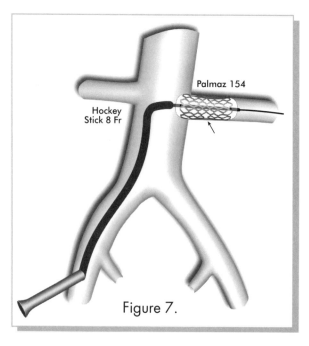

Palmaz 154

Hockey
Stick 8 Fr

Figure 7.

Figure 7. Stent deployment.

tion the stent at the lesion site. *(NB: Put negative pressure on the balloon catheter to prevent inadvertent inflation during contrast injections.)* For ostial lesions it is desirable to allow the stent to protrude several millimeters into the aorta, as the stent will shorten with expansion.

17. Deploy the stent with slow balloon inflation to 6 ATM. Inflate slowly to allow the balloon to develop a "dumb-bell" shape (**Figure 6**). This prevents asymmetric balloon inflation and possible stent embolization.

18. Withdraw balloon slightly so that the distal shoulder of the balloon is within the margins of the stent and inflate again to 8+ ATM (**Figure 7**). *(NB: This technique is helpful to "flare" the proximal stent in aorto-ostial lesions.)* Use contrast injections to judge the adequacy of deployment and reinflate the balloon to higher pressure, or select a larger balloon if necessary.

19. Remove the balloon and perform angiography to assess results.

VI. Assessing the results

1. Perform final angiography of the treated lesion.

    a. Assess stent expansion relative to the reference diameter.

        1) Generally, the there should be a slight over-expansion of the stent noted, ie. a "step-up and step-down" effect.

        2) If a significant (≥ 20%) diameter stenosis remains the lesion should be dilated with a larger balloon or at higher pressure. *(N.B. In a consecutive series of 100 patients, the only procedural variable that correlated with six month patency was a larger post-stent MLD.)*

    b. Determine that there is good distal run-off, without proximal or distal dissections to impair either inflow or outflow. If run-off is sluggish, search for its cause. Poor flow will jeopardize stent patency. If a flow-limiting dissection is discovered it should be treated with additional balloon inflations or a second stent.

2. Measure the translesional hemodynamic gradient.

   a. The final translesional gradient may be measured with either the post-dilation balloon or with an angiographic catheter across lesion.

   b. The gradient across the lesion should be less than 5 mmHg following stent placement.

3. Perform intravascular ultrasound (IVUS) imaging (optional). *(NB: Most IVUS systems will require that you exchange the 0.035-in wire for a 0.014-in guidewire.)*

   a. For optimal long-term patency the stent minimal lumen diameter (MLD) should be equal to or slightly larger than the reference vessel MLD.

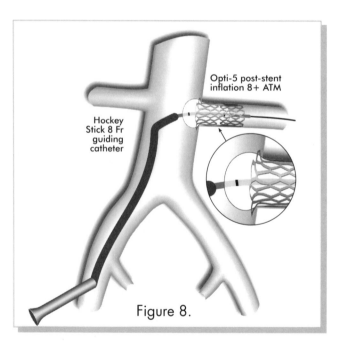

Opti-5 post-stent inflation 8+ ATM

Hockey Stick 8 Fr guiding catheter

Figure 8.

Figure 8. Flare the ostium of the stent with the balloon protruding into the aorta.

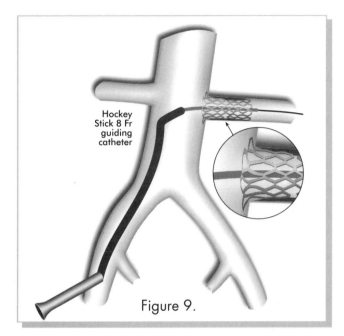

Figure 9. Note that the stent slightly pro- trudes into the aorta to ensure ostial coverage.

Hockey Stick 8 Fr guiding catheter

Figure 9.

b. The stent struts should be in contact with the vessel wall along the entire circumference of the vessel. If non-apposition of stent struts is identified, redilation with a larger balloon or at higher pressures is recommended.

c. The inflow and outflow portion of the stented segment should be carefully examined for evidence of a potentially flow-limiting dissection. Large dissections, or flow limiting dissections require treatment with additional balloon inflations or an additional stent.

VII. Sheath removal and follow-up care

1. Remove the sheath when the patient's ACT is ≤ 170 seconds.

2. Antihypertensive medications should be held until the immediate effect of renal artery reperfusion can be assessed (18 hrs to 24 hrs).

3. Patients are continued on aspirin indefinitely.

4. A follow-up visit at two to four weeks is appropriate to further adjust antihypertensive medications.

VIII. Lesion specific techniques

1. Aorto-ostial renal artery lesions are defined as those within 1 cm of the origin of the renal artery. This is the most common site of atherosclerotic lesions, and these lesions are historically difficult to treat with balloon dilation alone. The plaque is a continuation of aortic wall plaque, and significant recoil follows PTA alone.

    a. The stent should protrude slightly (1mm to 3 mm) into aorta. *(NB: Remember that the Palmaz stent will shorten during deployment. If the deployment is begun with the stent exactly at the ostium of the renal artery, the stent will shorten, thus uncovering the most proximal portion of the lesion.)*

    b. The ostium of stent should be flared with a high pressure balloon inflation. (**Figures 8 and 9**)

2. Multiple stent placement is required to correct either an error in the positioning of the original stent, or to cover a dissection.

    a. To recross the proximal stent, reinsert guiding catheter over a balloon so that the balloon-mounted stent is not at risk of catching on the original stent struts when advanced through the deployed stent.

    b. Overlap between the two stents should be minimized. Fortunately, the medium-sized Palmaz stents are readily visible on fluoroscopy which helps in positioning. *(NB: Remember to compensate for stent shortening during expansion.)*

IX. Troubleshootiing

1. **Pain with inflation:** Pain during balloon inflation should be taken as a warning of impending vascular rupture. When the patient experiences pain during inflation, the balloon should be immediately de-

flated and angiography performed to assess the condition of the dilated lesion.

2. **Tortuosity:** Severe vessel tortuosity or angulation can make renal stent deployment difficult. Wire position through the lesion should be gained with a flexible, steerable wire. The flexible wire may then be exchanged for a stiffer wire, which will help to straighten the tortuous vessel and allow more back-up support from the guiding catheter. Shorter length stents will negotiate bends more easily than longer stents.

3. **Incomplete stent expansion:** Incomplete stent deployment due to a pin-hole balloon leak is recognized when the indeflator will not hold pressure, and the stent is either undeployed, or underdeployed.
   a. Detach the 20 cc indeflator.
   b. Fill a 3 cc or 5 cc syringe with saline.
   c. Rapidly infuse saline (low viscosity) into the balloon, filling the balloon faster than the saline can leak out of the pin-hole, resulting in net balloon inflation and partial stent deployment.
   d. Withdraw the leaky balloon. If there is resistance within the stent, advance the guide catheter/sheath to be in contact with the stent, and pull the balloon into the guiding catheter.
   e. Replace the leaky balloon with new low-profile balloon and deploy the stent.

4. **Unable to predilate lesion:** The inability to fully expand a balloon during predilation is a contraindication to stent placement. *(NB: If the predilation balloon will not fully expand, placement of stent onto the balloon will not increase the ability of the balloon to dilate the lesion.)* Options are to abandon the stent procedure, or to use rotational atherectomy (Rotablator) to interrupt the constrictive band of fibrous tissue or calcification preventing complete balloon inflation.

5. **Recrossing stents:** To recross a deployed stent in the renal artery, a "J"

tipped guidewire should be used. Readvance the dilation balloon across the stent, and then place the guiding catheter/sheath over the balloon, and through the stent. The second stent may then be advanced distal to the first stent for deployment without risk of catching on the first stent.

6. **Stent embolization and retrieval**

   a. If the stent is pushed backwards off of balloon and onto the shaft of the balloon catheter the balloon should be withdrawn, and the stent remounted.

   b. If the stent is pushed off the front of the balloon and onto guidewire, care must be taken not to withdraw the guidewire. Attempts to remount the stent onto a new "lower profile" balloon may be carefully tried. If this fails, we recommend snaring the undeployed stent with a loop snare and pulling the stent back into the delivery sheath for removal.

      1) The loop snare is placed over the guidewire and advanced to the stent.

      2) The rearmost portion of the stent is secured in the snare, and the stent, the guiding catheter, and the guidewire are withdrawn as a single unit under fluoroscopic visualization to the femoral sheath.

      3) Once the stent is within the sheath, the sheath is removed over the guidewire, and then reinserted.

7. **Dissection:** If a flow-limiting or large dissection occurs distal or proximal to stent that is not relieved with balloon dilation, a second stent should be placed. In both instances it is necessary to place the guiding catheter into the deployed stent over a balloon to allow the second stent to pass through or overlap with the first stent.

RENAL STENT EQUIPMENT

Name	Company	Size	Length
Arterial/Venous Percutaneous Catheter Introducer Set			
Brite–tip	Cordis	5–8 Fr	11,23,35,45,55,90 cm
Flex	USCI	6,8 Fr	11,23 cm
Daig	Daig	5.5,7.5 Fr	90 cm
Pinnacle	Medi–tech	5,6,7,8 Fr	10,25 cm
Ansel Flexor Check–Flo	Cook	6,7 Fr	45 cm
Ansel Flexor Tuohy	Cook	6,7 Fr	55 cm
Angiography Catheters			
Pigtail, IMA, Cobra, JR4, others	Various	4–6 Fr	~ 65–110 cm
Interventional Guiding Catheters			
Renal Standard, Renal Short, Hockey Stick, Multipurpose	Various	6–8 Fr	55 cm (Multipurpose 100 cm)
Renal Long (Guider Soft Tip)	Medi–tech	6–8 Fr	55 cm
Guidewires and Glidewires			
J–wire, Amplatz extra–stiff, Bentson, Rosen, others	Various	.035 in	~145–260 cm
Wholey	Mallinckrodt	.035 in	145,260 cm
Flex–T	Mallinckrodt	.018 in	135 cm
Storq	Cordis	.035 in	180,300 cm
SV	Cordis	.018 in	180,300 cm
Jindo	Cordis	.035–.022 in (taper)	145,180,300 cm
Roadrunner extra support	Cook	.018 in	180,270,300 cm
Nimble Glidewire	Cook	.035 in	145,180,260 cm
Nimble Floppy	Cook	.035 in	145,180 cm

77

RENAL STENT EQUIPMENT

Name	Company	Size	Length
PTA Dilatation Catheters			
Marshal	Medi–tech	4–8 mm x 1.5,2 cm	75,90,135 cm
Talon	Medi–tech	4–7 mm x 1.5,2 cm	90,135 cm
Blue–Max	Medi–tech	4–7 mm x 2 cm	75,120 cm
Ultra–Thin Diamond	Medi–tech	4–7 mm x 1.5,2 cm	75,120,135 cm
Opta LP	Cordis	4–8 mm x 2 cm	65, 80,110,135 cm
Powerflex plus	Cordis	4–8 mm x 2 cm	65,80,110,135 cm
Jupiter	Cordis	4.5–6 mm x 2 cm	80,120,155 cm
Pursuit	Cook	4–10 mm	80,120 cm
Stents			
Palmaz Medium	Cordis	4–9 mm	10,15,20 mm
Corinthian IQ	Cordis	4–8 mm	12,18,20 mm
Bridge X3 Biliary Plus	Medtronic AVE	5,6,7 mm	17 mm
Bridge Extra Support Biliary Plus	Medtronic AVE	5,6,7 mm	10,17 mm

Chapter Four

CAROTID ARTERY STENT PLACEMENT

Carotid Artery Stent Placement

I. Indications for carotid stent placement

1. Symptomatic or asymptomatic patients who meet clinical criteria for carotid endarterectomy for stenotic lesions ($\geq 70\%$ diameter stenosis) and one of the following (**Table 1 and 2**):

2. Technical limitations:
   a. Intracranial or intrathoracic location of the carotid lesion.
   b. Prior radiation therapy to the surgical field.
   c. Restenosis after carotid endarterectomy.

3. Comorbid conditions increasing the risk of surgery (ie: critical coronary lesions).

4. Patient's refusal of surgery.

5. Participation in a randomized trial comparing endarterectomy versus stent.

Table 1. Clinical Indications for Carotid Endarterectomy

- Symptomatic lesions (NASCET)
  > 50% diameter stenosis

- Asymptomatic lesions (ACAS)
  > 60% diameter stenosis

Table 2. Contraindications to Carotid Stent Placement

- Total occlusion.

- Thrombus containing lesion.

- Excessive vessel tortuosity.

- Severe contrast allergy.

- Intolerant of both aspirin, ticlopidine, or clopidogrel.

- Undilatable carotid lesion.

II. Performing diagnostic carotid angiography

1. Choosing a vascular access site
   a. Femoral artery access: This is the preferred site from which to perform ascending aortic arch angiography and 4 vessel cerebral angiography.
   b. Brachial artery access: This access is preferred when femoral artery access is not available due to occlusive ilio-femoral disease.
2. Diagnostic aortic arch and 4 vessel angiography (**Figure 1**).

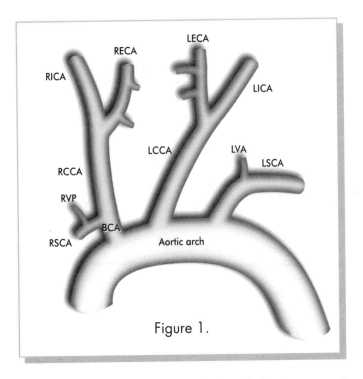

Figure 1.

Figure 1. Aortic arch vessels (BCA = brachial cephalic (innominate) artery, RVA = right vertebral artery, RCCA = right common carotid artery, RECA = right external carotid artery, RICA = right internal carotid artery, LCCA = left common carotid artery, LECA = left external carotid artery, LICA = left internal carotid artery, LVA = left vertebral artery, LSCA = left subclavian artery.

a. Postion the 6 Fr pigtail catheter proximal to the take-off the innominate artery.

b. Perform cineangiography with a 9-inch or larger image intesifier at 12.5 frames/sec to 15 frames/sec in a 30° to 60° LAO projection. *(NB: LAO angulation allows optimal visualization of the origins of the arch vessels.)*

c. Use a low osmolar, low viscosity, ionic contrast (Hexabrix-320) or non-ionic contrast for angiography.

CHAPTER FOUR: CAROTID ARTERY

d. The injection rate, using a power injector, is from 20 cc to 25 cc per second for 2 or 3 seconds.

e. Pan the table to visualize the cranial vessels as needed.

f. Subtraction angiography of the aortic arch provides better resolution and visualization of the arch vessels by subtracting the bony elements. Lower rates of contrast injections (15 cc to 20 cc over 1 sec to 2 sec) may be used. The limitation of this technique is that it does not allow panning of the field of view.

3. Selective common carotid angiography

a. Right common carotid artery: Selectively engage the innominate artery with a with a 6 Fr Judkins right coronary catheter.

1) Identify the origin of the right common carotid artery with test injections of contrast.

2) Advance a Wholey wire (0.035-in steerable wire) into the common carotid artery and advance the Judkins catheter over the wire.

3) Perform hand injections of 8 cc to 10 cc contrast.

b. Left common carotid artery: Depending on the origin of the left common carotid artery a number a catheters are available for selective cannulation of this vessel. Usually, the 6 Fr Judkins right coronary catheter can engage this vessel. Other useful catheter shapes include the Headhunter I & II, the internal mammary, or the Simmons (Shepherd's crook shapes) I, II or III.

1) Engage the origin of the left common carotid artery and confirm the catheter position with test injections of contrast.

2) The diagnostic catheter may be advanced several centimeters into the vessel over a J-tipped 0.035-in guidewire to ensure a stable position.

3) An optional step at this point is to exchange the catheter that gained access for a multipurpose catheter with sideholes to reduce the risk of trauma or dissection during contrast injections.

 c. Perform cineangiography or subtracted views of the common carotid, internal and external carotid in the AP and lateral views using hand injections of low osmolar ionic (Hexabrix-320) or non-ionic contrast. *(NB: It is necessary to adjust the angulation to optimize the separation of the internal and external carotid arteries to more clearly define the lesion.)*

 d. It is important that the intracranial distributions of the cerebral arteries, including the Circle of Willis, be visualized in both the AP and lateral views to determine the baseline circulation and to look for intracranial vascular lesions.

III. Preparation for carotid artery stent placement

1. Premedicate the patient with 325 mg of aspirin daily, and PLAVIX (clopidogrel) 75 mg QD for several days prior to the planned procedure.

2. Anticoagulate the patient with 10,000 U of heparin, with additional heparin given as needed to maintain the ACT > 250 seconds.

3. Optional placement of a temporary right ventricular pacemaker may be used when the lesion involves the carotid bulb to compensate for the potential bradycardia following balloon inflation. Alternatively, some operators pretreat the patient with atropine 0.5 mg to prevent bradycardia.

4. Selection of stent delivery catheters will depend on the stent choice and vascular access location.

a. Femoral access: A multipurpose shaped coronary guide catheter is the catheter of choice to deliver stents. An 8 Fr guiding catheter will deliver the medium Palmaz stent (104, 154, or 204) while a 9 Fr guiding catheter or 7 Fr sheath is required for the Wallstent.

b. Brachial access: A more angulated guiding catheter is necessary to enter the common carotid arteries from the brachial approach. Simmons, internal mammary, Judkins right, and headhunter shapes may be helpful.

c. Direct common carotid puncture: For internal carotid lesions, access directly into the common carotid artery is an optional approach for experience operators. Direct Seldinger puncture of the carotid artery is performed and short sheath (6 Fr for medium Palmaz stents, and 7 Fr for Wallstents) is placed in the vessel. *(NB: The potential complication of a large hematoma which can embarrass airway patency requires exceptional care with this approach.)*

IV. Technique for common carotid artery stent placement

1. Engage the common carotid with a 6 Fr diagnostic catheter of choice and confirm that the ACT is > 250 seconds.

2. Advance an exchange length 0.035-in Wholey wire or an extra-support 0.014-in angioplasty wire across the lesion and into the external carotid artery.

3. Perform baseline angiography of the target lesion.

4. Measure the reference diameter and length of the lesion.

5. Mark the lesion with bony landmarks or an external radiopaque ruler.

6. Exchange the diagnostic catheter for a guiding catheter/sheath (8 Fr or 9 Fr) and advance the guiding catheter/sheath to the proximal portion of the common carotid artery.

7. Predilate the lesion with a 4 mm x 40 mm low profile balloon to minimize trauma and decrease the risk of distal emboli when crossing the lesion.

    a. Inflate the balloon to the lowest pressure that results in complete balloon expansion for ≤ 10 seconds.

    b. Quickly deflate and remove the balloon, leaving the guidewire across the lesion.

    c. Perform angiography to assess the results of balloon angioplasty (ensure adequate predilation and to look for distal dissection).

8. Palmaz stent placement: For vessels ≤ 9 mm in diameter a medium Palmaz stent (104,154, or 204) long enough to cover the lesion is mounted on a balloon size 1:1 with the reference vessel diameter. For common carotid arteries > 9 mm a large Palmaz stent (188 or 308) will be required.

    a. Advance the balloon-mounted Palmaz stent to the lesion site, taking care that it does not catch on calcium in the lesion as it crosses the predilated lesion.

    b. Once the position of the stent has been confirmed, rapidly inflate the balloon to 6 ATM for several seconds, then deflate, and withdraw the balloon into the guiding catheter.

9. Wallstent deployment: A Wallstent is selected whose nominal diameter is at least 1 mm larger than the reference vessel, and whose length will cover the lesion.

    a. Advance the Wallstent over the guidewire and through the 9 Fr guiding catheter to the target lesion in the common carotid artery.

b. Placement of the stent is guided by either bony landmarks, an external ruler, or contrast injections through the arterial sheath or guiding catheter.

c. Advance the Wallstent several centimeters above the target lesion, and withdraw the sheath membrane about one-quarter of its length. The Wallstent may be pulled back, but not advanced once the stent has begun to expand, so the operator should err on the side of distal placement, and make subsequent adjustments by withdrawal in small increments. *(NB: It is possible to reconstrain the stent within the constraining sheath if the "point of no return" marked with a radiographic marker on the shaft of the delivery catheter has not been exceeded.)*

d. With the Wallstent in the appropriate position, the sheath is completely withdrawn to fully deploy the stent.

10. Reinsert the predilation balloon so that the distal shoulder of the balloon is within the stent and perform a high pressure (8+ ATM) inflation.

11. Perform final angiography.

V. Technique for internal carotid artery stent placement

1. Gain venous access for placement of a temporary pacemaker.

   a. Prophylactic placement of the pacemaker is optional, but it should be readily available if needed.

   b. Most patients are adequately protected from severe bradycardia by pretreatment with atropine.

2. Obtain arterial access and engage the common carotid artery with a 6 Fr diagnostic catheter of choice and confirm the ACT is > 250 seconds (**Figure 2**).

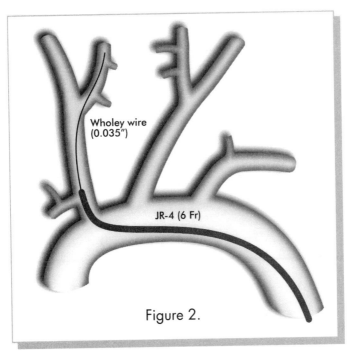

Figure 2.

Figure 2. Engage the ostium of the innominate artery with a 6 Fr Judkins right-4 diagnostic catheter. Advance an 0.035-in Wholey wire into the external carotid artery.

3. Perform baseline angiography to optimize the view of the target lesion. It is also recommended that if not already obtained, baseline views (AP & LAT) of the intracerebral vessels be obtained for later reference.

4. An 0.035-in exchange length Wholey wire is advanced into the *external* carotid artery and the 6 Fr. diagnostic catheter is advanced into the common carotid artery (**Figure 3**). In very tortuous vessels, it is advisable at this time to exchange the Wholey wire for a rigid, Amplatz extra-stiff wire to aid trackability of the guiding catheter into the common carotid artery (**Figure 4**).

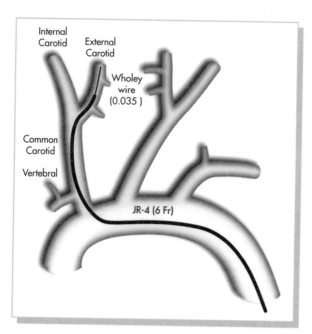

Figure 3. Advance the diagnostic catheter over the Wholey wire into the external carotid artery.

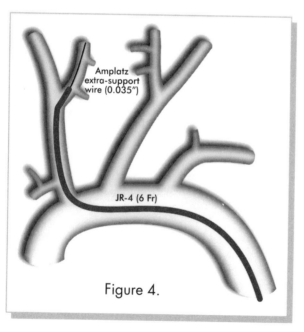

Figure 4.

Figure 4. Replace the Wholey wire with an 0.035-in extra-stiff Amplatz wire.

Figure 5. Exchange the diagnostic catheter for a 9 Fr multipurpose guiding catheter or 7 Fr Cook Sheath, to the common carotid artery.

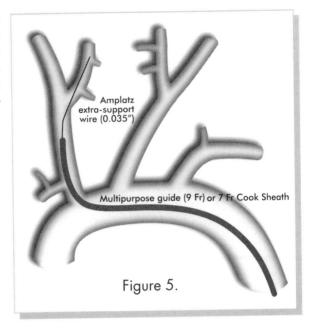

Figure 5.

Figure 6. Exchange the Amplatz wire for an 0.014-in extra-support angioplasty guide-wire and advance this wire across the lesion in the internal carotid artery.

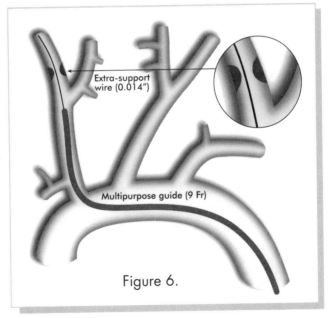

Figure 6.

5. Exchange the 6 Fr. diagnostic catheter for either an 8 Fr or 9 Fr multipurpose shaped coronary guiding catheter (**Figure 5**).

6. Measure the reference vessel diameter and lesion length.

7. Withdraw the 0.035 guidewire from the external carotid and cross the *internal* carotid lesion with a 0.014-in or 0.018-in stiff bodied coronary guidewire (**Figure 6**). *(NB: Take care to keep the distal wire below the carotid siphon to avoid vascular spasm and wire dissections in this tortuous segment of the vessel.)*

8. Select a 4.0 mm diameter and 40 mm long coronary balloon to predilate the lesion (**Figure 7**).

   a. The extra-long balloon prevents movement of the balloon (watermelon seeding) during predilation.

   b. Atropine 0.5 mg should be administered prior to balloon inflation to blunt the reflex bradycardia frequently seen.

   c. Inflate the balloon to ensure full expansion and deflate quickly. *(NB: many patients will experience significant bradyarrythmias and hypotension during balloon inflation.)*

9. Placement of a Palmaz stent: Using the reference diameter measurements for the internal carotid artery, select an appropriately sized balloon to mount a medium sized Palmaz stent (104, 154, or 204) (**Figure 8**). *(NB: There have been reports of external compression of balloon expandable stents at this location.)*

   a. Hand crimp the stent onto the balloon and advance it to the *internal* carotid lesion site.

   b. Care must be taken not to have the bare stent catch on plaque elements of the predilated lesion when crossing the lesion.

   c. Confirm the position of the stent and rapidly inflate the balloon to 6 ATM for several seconds, rapidly deflate the balloon, and withdraw the balloon into the guiding catheter.

Figure 7.
Predilate the
lesion with a
c o r o n a r y
angio-plasty
balloon.

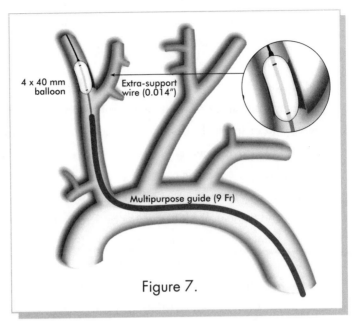

Figure 7.

Figure 8.
Deploy a
Palmaz stent
at the lesion
site.

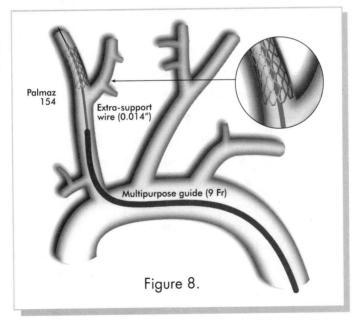

Figure 8.

d. If it is necessary to place a second stent in common carotid artery, repeat the above sequence with a larger balloon sized for the common carotid artery.

10. Placement of a Wallstent: A Wallstent is selected whose nominal diameter is at least 1 mm larger than the reference vessel (common carotid or internal carotid), and whose length will cover the lesion. *(NB: We currently use either 8mm or 10mm diameter Wallstents for all lesions at the bifurcation.)*

a. The Wallstent is advanced over the 0.014-in or 0.018-in guidewire and through the 9 Fr guiding catheter to the target lesion. Placement of the stent is guided by either bony landmarks, an external ruler, or contrast injections through the arterial sheath or guiding catheter *(NB: There is significant danger of air injections due to the tight fit of the Wallstent in the guide catheter which prevents brisk backbleeding to clear the guiding catheter).*

b. The Wallstent is advanced several centimeters above the target lesion, and the sheath membrane is withdrawn about 1/4 of its length (**Figure 9**). The Wallstent may be pulled back, but not advanced once the stent has begun to expand, so the operator should err on the side of distal placement, and make subsequent adjustments by withdrawal in small increments. *(NB: It is possible to reconstrain the stent within the constraining sheath if the "point of no return" marked with a radiographic marker on the shaft of the delivery catheter has not been exceeded.)*

c. With the Wallstent in the appropriate position, the constraining membrane is completely withdrawn to fully deploy the stent (**Figure 10**).

Figure 9.
Withdraw the con-straining sheath to de-ploy the Wallstent.

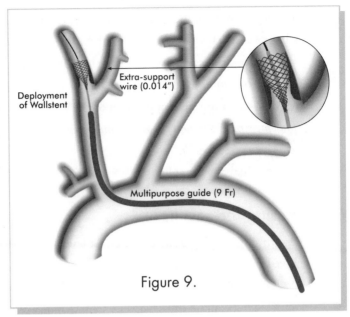

Deployment of Wallstent

Extra-support wire (0.014")

Multipurpose guide (9 Fr)

Figure 9.

Figure 10.
Completely deploy the Wallstent.

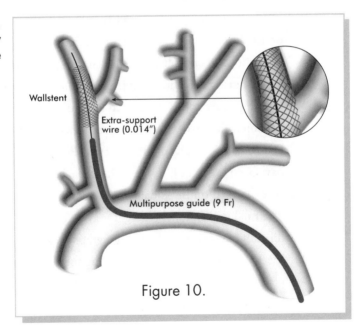

Wallstent

Extra-support wire (0.014")

Multipurpose guide (9 Fr)

Figure 10.

CHAPTER FOUR: CAROTID ARTERY

11. Post-deployment of the Wallstent or Palmaz stent is performed with a balloon sized 1:1 with the diameter of the internal carotid artery. The balloon is positioned so that the distal shoulder of the balloon is within the stent to avoid distal dissections. The balloon may be inflated to 8+ ATM to ensure stent apposition to the vessel wall. *(NB: We avoid "high pressure" inflations if possible and accept ≤ 20% residual diameter stenosis as a final result.)*

12. Perform final angiography.

VI. Assessing the results

1. Perform final angiography of the target lesion with the guidewire removed for lesion assessment.

   a. Assess stent expansion relative to the distal reference diameter. If a significant (≥ 30%) diameter stenosis remains the lesion should be dilated either with a larger balloon or at higher pressure.

   b. Determine that there is good distal run-off, and no proximal or distal dissection of vessel has occurred to impair either inflow or outflow. If run-off is sluggish, search proximally and distally for its cause. Poor flow will jeopardize stent patency. If a flow-limiting dissection is discovered it should be treated with either balloon inflations or a second stent if necessary.

   c. Perform angiography of the intracranial vessels to insure that there have been no emboli to the intracranial vessels or distal spasm.

2. Measure the final translesional hemodynamic gradient (optional).

   a. The final translesional gradient may be measured with the post-dilation balloon or with an angiographic catheter across lesion.

   b. Ideally, the gradient across the lesion should be resolved with stent placement. It is acceptable to terminate the procedure, however, once the gradient has been reduced to less than 5 mmHg.

VII. Sheath removal and post-procedure care

1. Remove the vascular sheath when the ACT is ≤ 170 seconds.
2. Perform a careful neurological examination following the procedure before arterial sheath removal and also prior to discharge.
3. Perform carotid duplex imaging of the stented segment as a baseline examination for comparison with future examinations.
4. Discharge the patient when stable, usually within 24 - 36 hours of the stent procedure on daily aspirin, 80 mg to 325 mg indefinitely, and Plavix (clopidogrel) 75mg once a day for 4 weeks.

VIII. Lesion specific techniques

1. **Ostial lesions:** Ostial common carotid artery lesions are intrathoracic, therefore not subject to external compression. They require a high degree of precision for optimal placement. The Palmaz medium stent is preferred in this location.

    a. Engage the ostium of the target vessel with a 6 Fr diagnostic catheter to minimize catheter trauma (usually a Judkins right-4, Headhunter, or Internal mammary shape) and perform baseline angiography of the lesion. Quantitative measurements are made to determine the size of the reference vessel.

    b. Cross the lesion with an exchange length, 0.035-in steerable wire (Wholey). Exchange the diagnostic catheter for an 8/9 Fr multipurpose coronary guiding catheter.

    c. Predilate with a balloon sized 1:1 with the reference vessel. During deflation of the balloon, advance the guiding catheter over the balloon and across the lesion. *(NB: Placing the guiding catheter across the lesion allows the stent to be advanced to the lesion without risk of dislodgement.)*

97

d. Mount a medium-sized Palmaz stent on the predilation balloon and advance it within the guiding catheter to the lesion site. Pull the guide catheter back using contrast injections to aid in precise stent positioning. Position the stent so the that it protrudes several millimeters proximal to the lesion (the stent will shorten 10 to 15 % during expansion). Deploy the stent by inflating the balloon to 6 to 8 ATM. If there is doubt about the location of the stent with regard to the ostium of vessel, IVUS may be helpful.

2. **Carotid bifurcation lesions:** Carotid bifurcation lesions are one of the most common lesions treated. Because the stent must make a transition from the smaller internal carotid to the larger common carotid artery, the self-expanding Wallstent (sized 1 mm larger than the common carotid artery) is generally the stent of choice.

3. **Intracranial lesions:** These lesions usually occur in tortuous segments of the carotid artery, and require a delicate touch and extreme control over guidewire movements to prevent distal dissections. The reference vessel diameter is 3 mm to 4 mm. Coronary balloons and stents are commonly used.

4. **Ulcers and thrombus:** Ulcerated lesions and those with angiographic thrombus are at high risk for embolization and are not generally suitable for stent placement. Thrombus-containing lesions should be pretreated for days to weeks with anticoagulants and reapproached after the thrombus has resolved.

5. **Occlusions:** Carotid occlusions are not candidates for recanalization due to the embolic risk associated with the procedure.

6. **Bilateral lesions:** Bilateral carotid lesions should not be treated sequentially in one procedure but staged over 2 procedures. In general, the most severe lesion should be treated first. If bilateral lesions are treated there is increased risk of a "hyperperfusion" syndrome.

IX. Troubleshooting

1. **Tortuosity:** Severe vessel tortuosity can make access and carotid stent deployment very difficult. Options include the use of progressively more stiff guidewires to facilitate tracking of the guiding catheter. *(NB: Tortuous lesions are associated with a higher complication rate than straightforward lesions, and should only be approached by experienced operators.)*

   a. If unable to advance a guiding catheter into a severely angulated carotid artery, one option is to place a Wallstent without a guiding catheter using bony landmarks for reference. Small amounts of dilute contrast can be injected through the sheath lumen to guide placement.

   b. One option for carotid stent placement complicated by a tortuous aorta or iliac artery disease is to perform the procedure from the brachial artery.

   c. Another option is to perform a direct carotid puncture for access, and to perform the procedure through a short sheath. This technique requires experienced hands and has the risk of a serious hematoma after sheath removal.

2. **Bradycardia and hypotension:** Transient bradycardia and hypotension are very common during carotid bifurcation stenting. Treatment with atropine, a temporary pacemaker, or both may be required. Occaisionally, prolonged (12 hrs to 36 hrs) hypotension occurs which is treated with a neosynephrine infusion titrated to the blood pressure response.

3. **Embolic events:** Intracerebral emboli may be detected by post-procedural neurological examination or on post-procedural intracerebral angiography (compared to the baseline intracerebral images). These emboli are either thrombi or plaque elements. Treatment consists of vasodilators, selective administration of urokinase, or balloon dilation to restore flow. *(NB: This complication requires a skilled operator with neuroradiologic experience. It is desirable to have a neuroradiologist available for consultation and assistance should this complicaton occur.)*

4. **Dissections:** Internal carotid artery dissections (flow-limiting) distal to the stent may be treated with balloon dilation to "tack up" the flap or with additional stent placement.

5. **Contralateral occlusions:** Contralateral carotid artery occlusions markedly increase the risk and difficulty of the procedure. They require rapid inflation and deflation of balloons during the procedure, and may be associated with seizures during balloon inflation.

CAROTID STENT EQUIPMENT

Name	Company	Size	Length
Arterial/Venous Percutaneous Catheter Introducer Set			
Brite–tip	Cordis	6,7,8,9 Fr	90 cm
Flex	USCI	8,9 Fr	11 cm
Shuttle–SL Flexor	Cook	6,7,8 Fr	90 cm
Angiography Catheters			
VTK	Cook	5 Fr	125 cm
Pigtail, Multipurpose, IMA, Simmons (1,2,3), Headhunter (1,2), others	Various	6 Fr	110 cm
Interventional Guiding Catheters			
Multipurpose, JR 4, others	Various	8,9 Fr	98 cm
Carotid Tuohy Borst Set	Cook	7 Fr	90 cm
Burke, H1, HY1, MPC, MPD	Cordis	8,9 Fr	95 cm
Guidewires			
J–wire, Amplatz, Bentson	Various	.035 in	~145–260 cm
Wholey	Mallinckrodt	.035 in	145,260 cm
Glide, angle (reg/stiff)	Medi–tech	.035 in	180,260 cm
Platinum–plus	Medi–tech	.014 in	180,260 cm
Storq	Cordis	.035 in	180,300 cm
SV	Cordis	.018 in	180,300 cm
Flex–T	Mallinckrodt	.018 in	135 cm
Loc Wire	Mallinckrodt	.035 in	200 cm
Extra–support	Guidant	.014 in	180,260 cm
Roadrunner	Cook	.018 in	180,270,300 cm

CAROTID STENT EQUIPMENT

Name	Company	Size	Length
PTA Dilatation Catheters			
Marshal	Medi–tech	4–10 mm x 1.5,2,3,4,6 cm	135 cm
Talon	Medi–tech	4–7 mm x 1.5,2,4 cm	135 cm
Blue–Max	Medi–tech	4–12 mm x 2,3,4 cm	120 cm
Ultra–Thin Diamond	Medi–tech	4–10 mm x 1.5,2,3,4,6 cm	120,135 cm
Opta LP (.035)	Cordis	4–10 mm x 2,4 cm	135 cm
Jupiter (.018)	Cordis	4.5–6 mm x 2,4 cm	120,155 cm
Savvy (.018)	Cordis	3–6 mm x 2,4 cm	120,135 cm
Ranger	Scimed	4 mm x 40 mm	135 cm
Stents			
Wallstent RP	Medi–tech	5–16 mm	20,40,60 mm
Palmaz medium	Cordis	4–9 mm	10,15,20 mm
Corinthian IQ	Cordis	4–8 mm	12,15,18,29,39 mm
Smart .018	Cordis	6–10 mm	20,30,40 mm

For additional

titles by

Physicians' Press

please be sure to visit

our bookstore at

www.physicianspress.com